CHI
HEALTH
CYCLE

To Bryon Fitzpatrick, my father-in-law, who was
always true to himself and dedicated to his art.

First published as *Clock On to Health* in Australia in 2019

Published by Welbeck Balance
An imprint of Welbeck Publishing Group Limited
20 Mortimer Street
London W1T 3JW

ISBN 978-1-78739-587-9

A CIP catalogue for this book is available from the British Library.

Printed in Spain

10 9 8 7 6 5 4 3 2 1

This book outlines a healthy lifestyle based on Traditional Chinese Medicine. A
healthy lifestyle supports all other forms of treatment.
It is not intended as a substitute for the medical advice of physicians. Always
consult health professionals in matters relating to health
and particularly in regards to any symptoms that may require
diagnosis or medical attention.

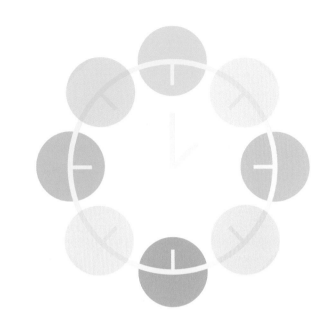

— CHI —
HEALTH
CYCLE

The 24-hour plan to restore
health through energy flow

JOST SAUER

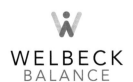

WELBECK
BALANCE

CONTENTS

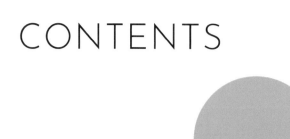

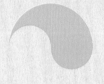

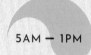

5AM — 1PM

INTRODUCTION 6

1. Thrive 12
The rhythm of health

PART 1 DRIVE 26

2. Large intestine 28
Out with the old
and in with the new

3. Stomach 38
Make peace not war

4. Spleen 48
Create your life

5. Heart 58
Rule your kingdom

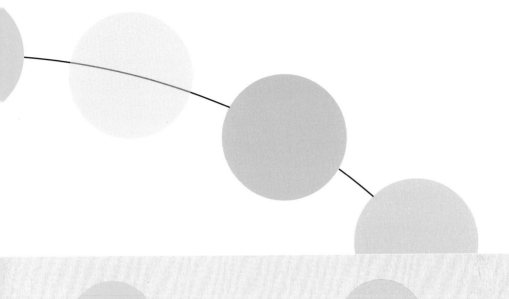

1PM — 9PM

PART 2 CRUISE   68

6. Small intestine   70
Make the right decisions

7. Bladder   82
Take the road to health

8. Kidneys   90
Pull your own strings

9. Pericardium   100
Protect your soul

9PM — 5AM

PART 3 SNOOZE   112

10. San jiao   114
Journey to the mystical

11. Gallbladder   122
Bring your 'A' game

12. Liver   132
Lead yourself to victory

13. Lungs   142
Act with honour

Conclusion   156
Index   157
Acknowledgements   160

INTRODUCTION

To be skilled at nurturing one's nature is to treat disease before it arises.
SUN SIMIAO

We are in the midst of a modern health meltdown. Lifestyle diseases , the lifestyle-related preventable chronic diseases such as heart disease, obesity and Type 2 diabetes – kill as many as 40 million people every year. Anxiety, depression and loneliness are widespread, and dementia (including Alzheimer's disease) is manifesting in ever-younger demographics. It's time to make some healthy changes so we can all feel good again.

An unhealthy lifestyle is at the root cause of the health crisis. Stress, insufficient exercise, lack of sleep, poor diets and smoking and drinking are considered key contributors. Lifestyle medicine, a relatively new idea in Western health, has arisen in response. It recommends behavioural and lifestyle changes such as exercise, stress management and better nutrition. However, changing lifestyle habits to prevent illness and simultaneously promote health, happiness and a sense of purpose is integral to Traditional Chinese Medicine, and has been for thousands of years.

I was introduced to the idea of lifestyle as a preventative health strategy when I studied acupuncture, and was immediately intrigued. Prior to studying, I'd gone through a period of drug addiction and, during my self-driven recovery, had developed a daily routine that slowly restored my health and happiness. The key components were exercise, nutritious foods, supplementation, living with purpose and tai chi. Studying Traditional Chinese Medicine not only made me realize that I'd prototyped my own modern medicinal lifestyle, but it also enabled me to improve it.

Traditional Chinese Medicine works with the 24-hour flow of chi (qi) through the body and the healing power of the organs. Every 24 hours chi spends two hours in each of the 12 organs. I discovered that every hour has a purpose and that if I synced certain activities with chi flow to the organs, it amplified health and happiness. I spent years experimenting and researching, and then created the chi cycle routine, a set of guidelines that restructures the day based on the very best times for everything.

It's not just lack of exercise, poor diet and stress that makes for an unhealthy lifestyle, it is also what you do when. If your day goes against the body's natural rhythms, it causes chi stagnation and physical and emotional pain. The chi cycle routine reverses this. It changed my life and I've seen it create great results for my clients in treating everything from addiction issues (my early area of specialization) to anxiety, depression, panic disorders and lifestyle disease.

The best part is that you don't have to give everything up, just reschedule. For example, have your coffee after breakfast, not before, and you increase nutrient absorption and prevent bloating, snacking and weight gain. Exercise in the morning rather than in the evening and you burn fat faster and reduce blood pressure. Work hard in the morning rather than at night and you get more done in less time, plus you boost immunity and lose weight. Small percentage gains add up to major health improvements and you feel better every day.

In 2009, I wrote my first book on my discoveries: *The Perfect Day Plan*, and since then numerous readers have told me that over a period of time following the routine, they lost weight without dieting, slept better, felt happier and many symptoms such as bloating, acid reflux, anxiety, brain fog and constant tiredness simply vanished. Other symptoms – including high blood pressure, insomnia and chronic inflammation – were also alleviated. This is because the chi cycle routine activates the natural healing power of your organs.

In Traditional Chinese Medicine, every symptom imaginable can be identified as the logical outcome of a specific organ condition, which is almost always caused by lifestyle factors. Traditional Chinese Medicine recognizes 'patterns' of symptoms affiliated with particular organs, and that these patterns can be reversed through a lifestyle that prioritizes organ health. This book introduces a few basic concepts of Traditional Chinese Medicine, including yin and yang (see the glossary, overleaf), the 24-hour cycle of chi and nourishing your organs; it outlines how to use the chi cycle routine for self-treatment.

This is not a text book on Chinese medicine. I've simplified what I've learned from over 30 years of researching, teaching and practising Chinese medicine, and from using lifestyle therapeutically for my clients, into a lifestyle manual. It is a how-to guide you can use to take charge of your health and transform your life. It is lifestyle medicine inspired by ancient Chinese health secrets and designed for modern times.

GLOSSARY OF KEY TERMS

Chi

The energy that creates and sustains all life, chi flows through everything in the cosmos, in and around your body via its own network of meridians (the illustration below indicates the general location of 12 meridians). Chi is the basis for health and longevity. The flow of chi is regulated by yin and yang. If these forces are balanced, chi flows freely. Chi is the healing medium of Traditional Chinese Medicine.

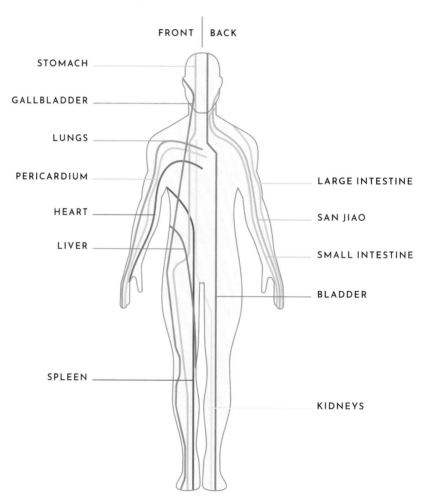

FRONT | BACK

STOMACH

GALLBLADDER

LUNGS

PERICARDIUM

HEART

LIVER

SPLEEN

LARGE INTESTINE

SAN JIAO

SMALL INTESTINE

BLADDER

KIDNEYS

Chi Cycle

Chi cycle is a term I use to describe the 24-hour flow of chi (qi) through the body. Aligning daily activities with this cycle promotes health, vitality and happiness.

Chi Practices

Tai chi and yoga are chi practices. They enable you to build and move chi yourself. Tai chi is a key self-healing modality of Traditional Chinese Medicine, and yoga is a key component of health in Ayurvedic medicine. They build your vital life force, enhance your blood flow, distribute oxygen and nutrients to your tissues, remove waste products from your arteries and reduce inflammation and stress. They also promote emotional and spiritual health as they lead to higher awareness. Both are based on the philosophy that there is order, beauty, harmony and purpose to all existence.

Meridians

The meridian system is a network of invisible chi pathways that map your body. There are 12 main meridians, each correlating to a limb and an organ. Acupuncture points are located on these meridians.

Yin and Yang

The concept of yin and yang, of duality forming a harmonious whole, is the basis of Chinese philosophy and medicine. Everything in nature consists of two interdependent and constantly shifting energies. Each contains an aspect of the other. Every 24 hours, yang (day/light) flows into yin (night/dark) in a universal cyclical movement. Yin and yang are also the basis for understanding health and for diagnosis. Imbalances (manifesting as yin or yang deficiencies or excess conditions) create illness and disease. Chinese medicine treatments work to restore balance.

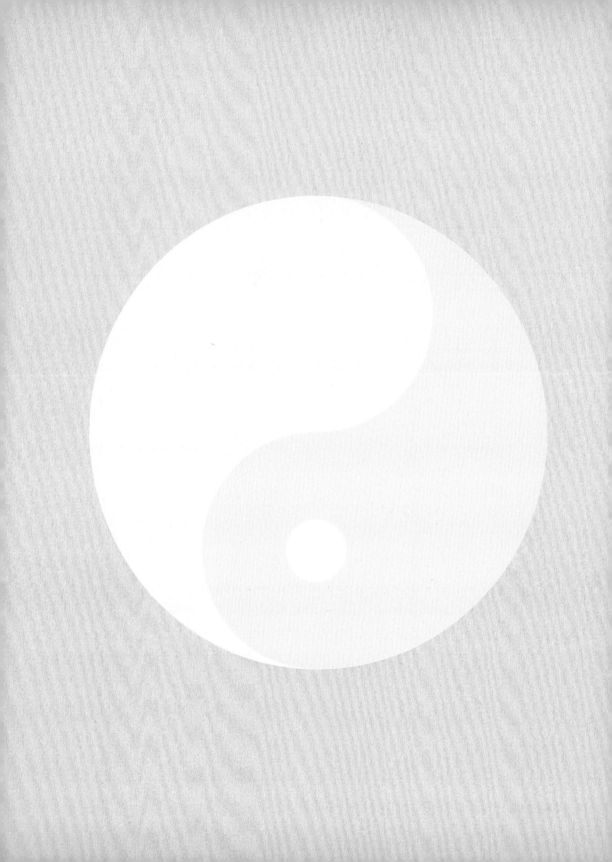

CHAPTER 1

THRIVE

THE RHYTHM OF HEALTH

Learning to align your daily activities with
chi flow to your organs will set you on the path
to health and vitality.

ACTIVATE YOUR OWN HEALING POWER

Health and happiness is your natural state. Your body has unlimited healing power and you can use your lifestyle to activate this – to heal yourself, become happy and have a fulfilling and peaceful life.

This is Traditional Chinese Medicine in a nutshell. It is one of the oldest medical systems, and it is natural and preventative. In Ancient China, physicians kept people well; if one of their patients became sick they would lose credibility and business. The patient had to do their part too, of course, by following a health-promoting lifestyle.

Traditional Chinese Medicine has been refining the art of healthy living ever since, but the fundamentals remain the same. You take responsibility for your health by living in a way that balances yin and yang, builds your chi (energy), and keeps chi flowing to all your organs.

Your organs are your personal disease-fighting and health-boosting team. If you give them lots of chi, they will heal symptoms and keep you healthy and happy.

LOVE YOUR ORGANS, LOVE YOUR LIFE

Traditional Chinese Medicine takes a very different approach to health to that of Western medicine. It is based on the understanding that everything you need to thrive physically, emotionally and spiritually is within you. Your organs are the stars of the show; they hold the secrets.

Your organs know how to heal you. It is, in fact, their job. Imagine them as your in-house specialists for physical, mental, emotional and spiritual health. You can put your trust in their expertise. If you care for your organs, your symptoms recede, your sense of wellbeing increases and your outlook improves. This, in turn, boosts your health. Life becomes a cycle of ever-increasing health and happiness.

Getting healthy shouldn't be a chore and it shouldn't mean depriving yourself of everything you enjoy. Follow the chi cycle routine and, as your chi builds, healthy new habits naturally replace unhealthy ones and the pursuit of health becomes a pleasure. This is a win-win health strategy.

MEET YOUR ORGAN TEAM

Western medicine treats the advanced stages of lifestyle diseases, but Traditional Chinese Medicine aims to stop things *before* they get serious. In Traditional Chinese Medicine, your organs have physiological functions similar to those of Western medicine, and in addition, each organ also has what you could describe as an 'energy organ' or 'chi organ' that has metaphysical functions.

Lifestyle diseases and illnesses begin with chi blockages and living in accordance with the chi cycle restores chi flow. Your organs will love this and you will too. When chi flows freely through your organs you feel great. How good you want to feel is up to you – with chi there are no limits.

I'm going to take you behind the scenes to meet your chi organs and discover how to use your lifestyle to nourish them. In Traditional Chinese Medicine there is no separation of body, mind and spirit – and its poetic language reflects this world view. Your heart, for example, is known as the Emperor, and your liver is the General. In this same spirit I've assigned roles to all your organs, to help you get to know them and understand the role they play in your health and happiness.

THE ORGANS AND THEIR ROLES

Large Intestine: The Cleaner

Stomach: The Peacemaker

Spleen: The Builder

Heart: The Emperor

Small Intestine: The Judge

Bladder: The Driver

Kidneys: The Puppeteer

Pericardium: The Bodyguard

San Jiao: The Ferryman

Gallbladder: The Coach

Liver: The General

Lungs: The Knight

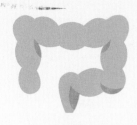

The Cleaner

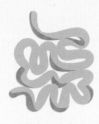

The Judge

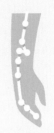

The Ferryman

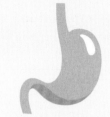

The Peacemaker

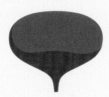

The Driver

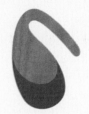

The Coach

The Builder

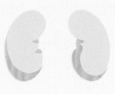

The Puppeteer

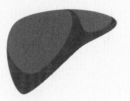

The General

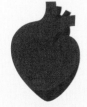

The Emperor

The Bodyguard

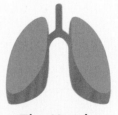

The Knight

LIVE YOUR LIFE TO A RHYTHM, NOT A SCHEDULE

Traditional Chinese Medicine works in harmony with daily, seasonal and even planetary cycles. An easy way to start improving your health is to get in sync with the daily flow of yin and yang (see page 11). These two opposite yet complementary forces cycle in harmony every 24 hours. In the morning yang ascends, peaking at midday; as yang begins descending, yin starts ascending. Yin peaks at midnight, and as it begins its descent, yang starts to ascend; the cycle continues.

THE THREE PHASES

At its simplest, your day is divided into three eight-hour phases that align with this flow: 'drive', 'cruise' and 'snooze'. In the morning, as yang gains momentum you do likewise by taking charge and driving your day until lunchtime. This builds chi. As the transition towards yin begins in the middle of the day you ease off the intensity and 'cruise' to keep chi flowing smoothly. Then in the evening, during the 'snooze' phase, the most yin part of the cycle, you back off completely and sleep.

This is the rhythm of health. Your organs follow this rhythm and the chi cycle routine enables you to live in harmony with it. None of us are supposed to be racing around day and night trying to keep up with crazy, over-committed schedules. That creates yin and yang imbalances and chi stagnation, which lead to uncomfortable symptoms, illnesses, and ultimately, disease. Follow the 'drive, cruise, snooze' rhythm instead and you'll be moving towards good health, vitality and happiness.

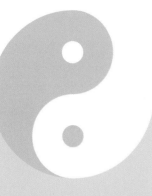

5AM — 1PM

DRIVE

Large intestine
Stomach
Spleen
Heart

In the morning, as yang gains momentum you take charge and 'drive' your day until lunchtime. This builds chi.

1PM — 9PM

CRUISE

Small intestine
Bladder
Kidneys
Pericardium

As the transition towards yin begins in the middle of the day you ease off the intensity and 'cruise' to keep chi flowing smoothly.

9PM — 5AM

SNOOZE

San jiao
Gallbladder
Liver
Lungs

In the evening, during the 'snooze' phase, the most yin part of the cycle, you back off completely and sleep.

THE TWO-HOUR TIME SLOTS

You can break each of the 'drive, cruise, snooze' phases down further into two-hour time slots and boost health benefits with some small life hacks. Chi flows through your body in a 24-hour cycle, spending two hours in each of your organs. If you realign normal daily activities – from sleep to social media – to the times that are most beneficial for specific organs, you will automatically enhance their function and your health.

Every symptom you have is associated with an organ. Back in Ancient China, you would be treated at the time chi was in that organ. These days no one's going to be turning up at 11pm to treat your gallbladder because you can't make decisions, or knocking on your door at 2am to treat your liver because you feel directionless, but they don't have to; follow the chi cycle routine and you will be treating your organs yourself throughout the day.

Small adjustments produce big improvements. Always wake up to 'drive' and finish with 'snooze'. Your organs respond to this rhythm. Align activities with the two-hour organ time slots when you can to amplify the health benefits still more.

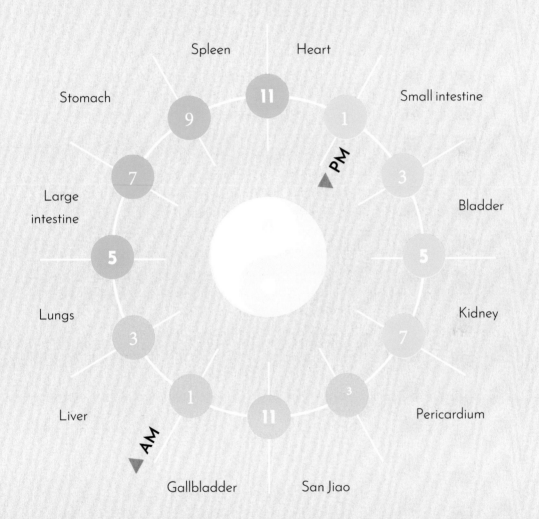

Spleen

Heart

Stomach

Small intestine

Large intestine

Bladder

Lungs

Kidney

Liver

Pericardium

Gallbladder

San Jiao

PM

AM

TREAT THE CAUSE
NOT THE SYMPTOM

Poor lifestyle choices have resulted in a modern health meltdown. Healthy choices are the solution. Lifestyle disease symptoms begin by the separation of yin and yang and chi stagnation, and health comes from living in a way that balances yin and yang and keeps chi flowing smoothly.

Day-to-day life naturally creates imbalances and stagnation, which manifest as common symptoms, ranging from aches and pains to mental or emotional imbalances. It is normal to have such symptoms but they are never random or accidental. Each is a logical outcome of a poor lifestyle choice. Traditional Chinese Medicine can join the dots from a seemingly unrelated, two-minute stressed-out breakfast to insomnia, and from there to heart disease. By the time a symptom becomes apparent, however, you will not make the connection to its original cause.

For example, if you are short of breath, you'll probably assume that it is a lung problem. But Traditional Chinese Medicine might see it as a spleen problem, because although your lungs store phlegm, which contributes to the shortness of breath, it is your spleen that creates phlegm. And your spleen does this as a result of a nutrient-poor diet, too much cold and raw food, or too much spicy and fatty food. But you might be eating those foods as a compensatory behaviour for another emotional or physical imbalance.

If you focus on one symptom and use a medication with a single active ingredient to try to treat it; it won't address the cause.

The chi cycle routine has what you could call multiple 'active ingredients'. Living in a healthy rhythm improves the function of all your organs simultaneously, and naturally changes the unhealthy behaviours that cause the symptoms. If you add Chinese herbal formulas, which always contain multiple active ingredients, and Traditional Chinese Medicine treatments that do likewise, you are on the track to health.

GETTING TO KNOW THE HEALTH RHYTHM

Familiarizing yourself with what your organs are up to throughout the day is a great start. You will slowly become more attuned to your organs and this alone will have a beneficial effect on your health. Get into a basic rhythm of being more active and productive in the first half of your day and more laid back in the second half. This will give you a feel for balancing yin and yang.

Make small changes to slowly sync with the health rhythm. Initially follow as much of the chi cycle routine as possible on your weekdays. You could enter the key daily activities into your weekly diary and start scheduling around them. Do whatever you like on weekends. After a while, you'll feel so much better on the chi cycle days that you will naturally want more of that at the weekend.

Don't become obsessed by the clock and get anxious if you miss an activity at its optimum time. Just keep the rhythm going. If you are a shift-worker, follow the 'drive, cruise, snooze' sequence regardless of what time it is. Always exercise when you wake up, and relax before you sleep. Your organs understand and respond to this routine.

NEW WAYS TO CHANGE

Balancing yin and yang might be a new idea for you, and you might
not have even heard of chi, but you are already working with both.
If you wake up tired, unable to face the day and have a couple of
coffees, you are getting yang up and setting off a chi flow. If you
come home wrecked after a long day and go for a bottle of wine
you are unwinding with yin; choose the break-up tub of ice-cream
and you are using chi flow to temporarily alleviate pain.

You are actually treating yourself all day in this way. The only
problem is that using food, drink or unhealthy behaviours compounds
the problem by intensifying the underlying chi stagnation and
imbalances. Symptoms pile up on one another and become worse,
with disease as the end result. At this point it is no longer possible
to change the way you feel with food, drink or unhealthy behaviours,
and that awful feeling of having run out of options takes hold.
Your outlook is bleak and life is no longer enjoyable.

The chi cycle routine introduces a sustainable way to change
the way you feel every two hours of the day. It is not an instant
cure, but as you start to live it, one day you'll suddenly realize that
a nagging symptom such as tiredness, bloating or thirst is gone.
Then you'll struggle to remember when it last bothered you.
At your next doctor's visit, they'll wonder why your blood pressure
is so much better. Stay in sync with the rhythm of health, and
soon you will notice another symptom has gone.

HOW TO USE THIS BOOK

The chapters for each phase relate to a particular organ, and each one sets out the healthy choices you can make to keep that organ in its best shape, and also reveals how the unhealthy choices that many of us unknowingly make create the symptoms that can progress to diseases. This is followed by tips for each time slot, suggesting good ideas as well as those that are not so good. At the end of each phase there is a summary of the time slots and what needs to happen during each one.

TREAT YOURSELF

The chi cycle routine enables you to treat your whole organ system continuously. It is a self-sustaining health and happiness system. It corrects the causes, treats existing symptoms, and prevents ill health from developing, while simultaneously helping you feel better every day. So you are treating yourself in every sense!

You can't imagine what your body is capable of, or how much better you can feel, until you start. And you can start immediately. It doesn't matter how unhealthy, unhappy or unwell you feel at this moment, just follow the flow of the health rhythm and change will happen. Drive then cruise through your days and snooze through your nights and you will thrive like never before!

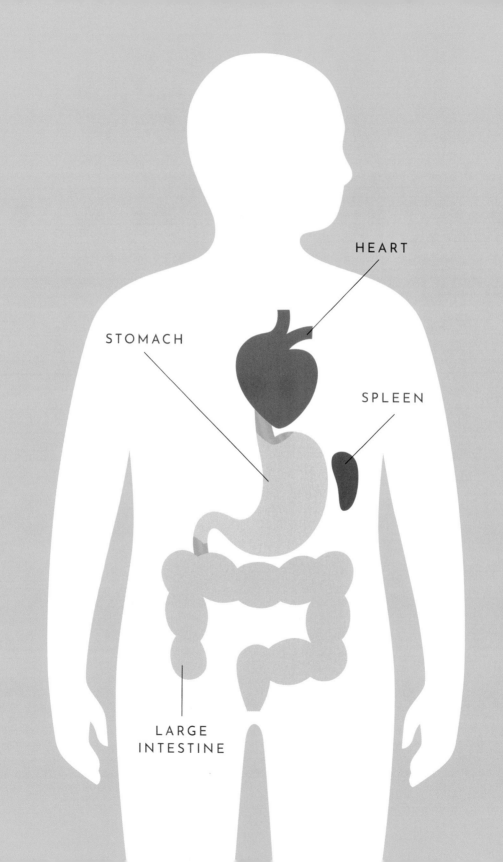

HEART

STOMACH

SPLEEN

LARGE
INTESTINE

DRIVE

5AM — 1PM

In the morning, as yang is building, the 'drive' phase begins.
In these eight hours your actions, food and intention build chi.
And the more chi you have, the happier and healthier you
can be. It's time to be proactive. Wake up and exercise, have
a calm breakfast, then work hard, following your life's purpose
and achieve goals, and you will build abundant chi.
You will also be aligned with the health rhythm of the day,
allowing chi to flow smoothly. All your organs will get what
they need to do a great job eliminating symptoms and
preventing more from developing. Remember that these
are your 'chi organs' we are talking about, and that all your
symptoms come from chi blockages or stagnation in the
meridians. Your organs are ready to go, so let's meet your
'drive' shift: the Cleaner (large intestine), Peacemaker
(stomach), Builder (spleen) and Emperor (heart).

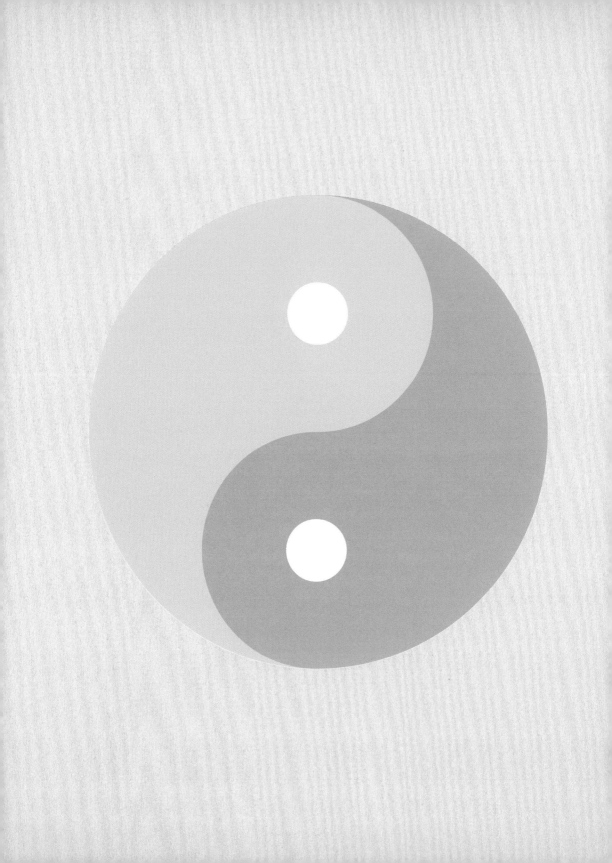

CHAPTER

2

LARGE INTESTINE

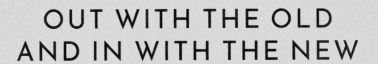

OUT WITH THE OLD
AND IN WITH THE NEW

First up is your large intestine. Each morning as the
clock strikes five, it is ready to eliminate all your old
physical and emotional waste. Meet the Cleaner.
This is the time to get up and exercise.

5AM — 7AM

HEALTHY CHOICES

GET UP AND EXERCISE

The Cleaner has two hours to work. To get the most out of its time and do the best cleaning job possible, get up as close to 5am as you can, drink some water, stretch and exercise (focusing on your core, glutes and thighs to boost energy and balance yin and yang in the body). This will lubricate your body with fluids, blood and chi.

These are your cleaning products, and the Cleaner will enthusiastically get to work. It hoses out your old emotional negativity, like that urge to get back at people who have said or done things that hurt you. It sweeps away your guilt over what you have said or done and later regretted; it vacuums up toxic stress and erases those annoying arguments that you have with people in your head.

Hydrate

Drinking some water in the morning is a small, easy change that will have a big impact on your health. If you don't usually drink water when you wake up, make it a new habit. It is essential for your health. Bodily fluids are concentrated while you sleep to prevent you from getting up to go to the toilet during the night. Water rehydrates your body, lubricates your joints (feeling stiff when you wake up can be due to dehydration), and enhances all your bodily functions.

Ideally you'd head for the bathroom next, as the water also flushes your organs, which will assist in evacuating your bowels. A regular bowel movement soon after waking is a sign of good health (dehydration is a factor in constipation).

Detox every morning

Your large intestine excretes waste products, and this includes negative emotions. In Traditional Chinese Medicine positive emotions are considered to be 'nutrients', and they are absorbed and used. Negative emotions are toxins, and morning exercise eliminates them, which helps prevent mental exhaustion.

The Cleaner also clears obstructions in your arteries and enhances your blood flow. This prevents the build-up of fat, cholesterol, calcium and other substances. The metaphysical clean extends to flushing out your meridians (the 12 invisible chi pathways in your body) to remove blockages before they can develop into physical symptoms.

Exercise early

If you exercise on an empty stomach, with nothing but water beforehand, energy will be drawn from stored fat. Toxins – the inflammatory elements from environmental, emotional or chemical sources – are stored in fat, so you'll be eliminating some potential contributors to high blood pressure, Type 2 diabetes, obesity and heart disease. You'll also lose weight. But keep your focus on exercising for large intestine health, rather than to lose weight – it will naturally contribute to sustainable weight loss.

Find at least 30 minutes to exercise, and you've made the most of the first opportunity of the day to put your health and happiness house in order. The Cleaner has done its job; you've let go of the old and can now move forward to the new in your life. This is a great thing to do for your physical and emotional health. It helps to ward off anxiety and depression.

Manage stress and prevent depression

If you start your day with exercises that give your core, glutes, and thighs a good workout, it builds strength and fitness and also activates acupuncture points that generate calmness and confidence (without the need for needles). This means you're not going to get as stressed during the day as you did before, even if someone sabotages or criticizes your work, micro-manages you or belittles your abilities or character.

You can't control the work environment or change other people's behaviour, but there are lots of little tricks, such as morning exercise, that you can use to reduce the negative emotional effects that people's words or deeds have on you. This applies not just at work, but with your partner, family or friends as well. It's worth the brief discomfort of some early morning exercise just to be able to access this. The weight loss, increased vitality and extra energy are welcome by-products.

This is the prime time for transformative change. Align with the health rhythm now, and the rest of your organ team can continue the good work of the Cleaner so you reap the benefits of your morning's effort all day long.

If you are retired, unemployed, work from home or don't have to rush through your morning, make the most of this health-boosting opportunity. Add a long walk, a yoga or tai chi class, a swim or a bike ride. Use the whole two hours and you will see significant improvements in your health.

UNHEALTHY CHOICES

The morning is your time of reckoning. The side-effects of your activities from the previous day, weeks or even years, are present as soon as you wake up. You may have aches and pains, feelings of anxiety, depression or low confidence, a dry mouth and/or throat, itchy skin, blurry vision, and/or feel generally unwell and unwilling to face the day.

Think of this as the rubbish that has been put out for the Cleaner. You'd never wake up and rummage through yesterday's trash, so don't lie in bed and think about, discuss or analyze how you feel. Just get up and move. Let the Cleaner take care of these symptoms.

Sleeping in

If you hit the snooze button instead, you make life hell for the Cleaner: you're sealing the windows shut so no fresh air can circulate. If you wake and immediately turn to social media, work or entertainment to distract yourself from how you feel, you're dumping more rubbish as fast as the old is being swept up. If you light up, grab a coffee or munch a sweet pastry, you're tracking mud all over the floors while the Cleaner is trying to mop. The Cleaner ends up doing a half-hearted swipe over the surfaces, while underneath the emotional and physical waste accumulates.

**Large intestine symptoms
When the trash piles up**

Physically, that internal mess impacts on all your organs. If the Cleaner can't do its job properly it affects how well all the other organs work, and contributes to a progression of symptoms that can eventually become a lifestyle disease.

Your organs affect your emotions and your emotions affect your organs. Unresolved anxiety, sadness or worry, in particular, can interfere with the functioning of your large intestine and create symptoms. A backlog of emotions can also encourage unhealthy behaviours. If you can't free yourself from people's negative comments or actions they can loop in your head and it is easy subconsciously to try to counter this negativity with something to make you feel good. For example, you might turn to comfort eating, which can lead to weight gain or Type 2 diabetes.

All your actions send messages to your organs. If you get up and exercise you are affirming that your health is your top priority and this conditions your organs to fight off disease. But if you wake and get straight into work or social media, or go for a cup of tea and the news, you are telling your organs that your health is not a priority. Symptoms are more likely to develop.

Even though any one symptom is connected to many organs in Traditional Chinese Medicine, there are what we call 'patterns', or sets of correlated symptoms, associated with specific organs. The symptoms affiliated with large intestine patterns include: abdominal pain, constipation/diarrhoea, dry mouth, loss of appetite, excessive thirst and mental exhaustion.

The good news is that all Traditional Chinese Medicine symptom patterns can be reversed. Making the healthy choices in these two hours conditions and improves the function of your large intestine and treats these symptoms. And you are also automatically helping all your other organs to function better and treating the symptom patterns affiliated with each of them. This is how the chi cycle routine targets the networks of symptoms that form lifestyle diseases.

Your organs affect your emotions and your emotions affect your organs.

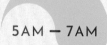

LIFESTYLE TIPS

DOS

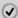

Use an alarm clock to wake up instead of your phone. Your mind is already going to come up with a number of excuses for you not to get up and having a digital device within reach makes it easier to give in.

Get a water filter. You need lots of water in the morning to rehydrate and get your energy moving and you don't want to be adding toxins with unfiltered water while your detox is underway.

Schedule your morning exercise so you know exactly what you are doing.

Buy yourself workout gear that you love and have it ready to put on, even if you are exercising at home.

Do a 'chi practice', such as yoga or tai chi, as well as other kinds of exercise.

If you meditate in the morning, be aware that meditation doesn't replace exercise.

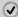

Include weight training three times a week. This is essential for a healthy body and healthy organs and is a key to ageing well. It lowers blood glucose levels, significantly lowering the risk of Type 2 diabetes, and it speeds up your metabolism.

Exercise whether you feel like it or not. Facing and overcoming resistance when you wake strengthens your willpower and motivation.

If you sleep in and/or don't have enough time for 30 minutes of exercise, do some stretching. If you do it every day it trains your organs and helps to form a new habit. You'll be more likely to feel like exercising, and less likely to listen to your mind trying to talk you out of it.

DON'TS

Avoid exercise because you feel awful when you wake up. The majority of people feel like that in the morning. Don't buy into this! It is just stagnation. Get moving, your chi will begin to move and you will instantly feel better.

Journal, vision or plan your life between 5am and 7am. This is toxin-elimination time, so journaling now is like heading to a rubbish dump to find inspiration for your life. Journal later – between 11am and 1pm is the best time, when chi is in your heart.

Lie in bed or sitting with a coffee or tea and thinking about your life. This is not a productive time for reflection. It can trap you in negative emotionality, which is not good for your health. You need to get moving, so chi flows, new options open up and your outlook becomes positive.

Have sex in the morning. It's common to wake up feeling sexually aroused, but this is energy mobilized for other purposes by your kidneys (which store your sexual energy). If you have sex now, you are using up the energy that you need to create your day.

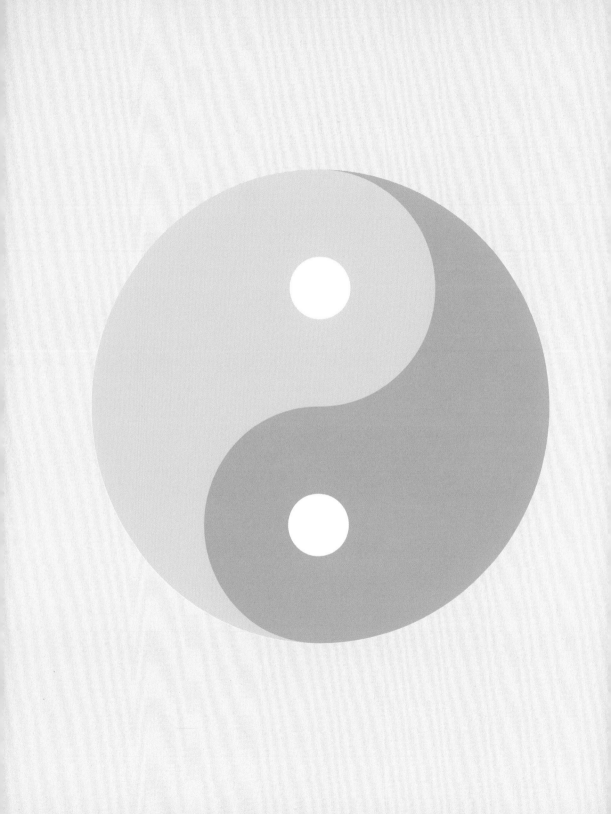

CHAPTER

3

STOMACH

MAKE PEACE
NOT WAR

As the clock strikes seven, chi moves to your stomach. Its job is to ensure that you have inner peace and a richly rewarding life. Your stomach is the Peacemaker. This is the time to eat a nutritious breakfast.

7AM — 9AM

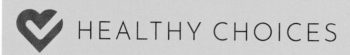

HEALTHY CHOICES

EAT A NUTRITIOUS BREAKFAST

The Peacemaker wants to make sure you start the day on good terms with yourself and others. All you have to do to enable it to do its job is take at least 20 minutes somewhere in this time slot to enjoy a peaceful and wholesome breakfast. If you have the right food (warm and nourishing), and eat it in the right way (mindfully, slowly and calmly), all will be well. So approach your breakfast imagining that a peace negotiation is underway, and your health and happiness depends on what and how you eat. It does.

Both what you eat and how you eat it trigger a chain reaction of organ processes that shape your body and your life. A healthy breakfast is more than a list of nutrients: it has to fill your stomach, taste good to make you feel good, and be eaten in peace. Your stomach is the centre of all chi pathways – 'chi central' – and if you get breakfast right, a sense of wellbeing infuses your entire body before you step out the door. This builds your blood, which is the foundation for health, and has a positive influence on everything that happens in the day ahead.

If you want to take charge of your health, always eat breakfast. Chi is in your stomach in the morning for a reason. You are about to go out into the day to create something – whether that is money, projects, support for your family or self-worth – and breakfast gives you the resources for this. It is also an important opportunity to balance yang with yin. If you consciously create the feeling that you have all the time in the world to eat (even if you don't), it builds yin and improves digestion. This is essential for health.

IDEAS FOR A NUTRITIOUS BREAKFAST

Your stomach was referred to as the 'keeper of the granaries' in the old medical books, and the Peacemaker likes to work with healthy grains. Here are some ideas for breakfasts that will infuse good feelings into your day.

- A delicious, creamy, oat porridge with roasted hazelnuts and natural cocoa powder (to add a chocolatey taste).
- Fluffy buckwheat pancakes drizzled with honey, toasted almonds and warmed blueberries.
- A steaming savoury congee made from rice or wholesome grains is considered a healthy breakfast in Traditional Chinese medicine as it nourishes the stomach.

Both what you eat and how you eat it trigger a chain reaction of organ processes.

Mindful eating

Lots of people assume that being healthy means going on an extreme diet or giving up grains and carbs. But nutritious grains are part of a healthy diet. It's the over-processed grains loaded up with sugar and fat (think sugary breakfast cereals or doughnuts) that you need to quit. If you are eating nutritious carbs or grains, changing the way you eat them will make all the difference. Don't rush! Be mindful of each mouthful, and after you finish breakfast take a few minutes to just sit calmly and do nothing. You probably think that you don't have time for that but ultimately it will save you time, because you will be more focused afterwards, which means your morning will be much more productive.

This kind of mindful breakfast helps you maintain a healthy weight. It enhances nutrient absorption and provides a feeling of satiation (you get attuned to this after a while) that naturally stops you overeating. Plus, you won't nibble your way through the morning. Constant snacking interferes with the Peacemaker's job; it requires a rhythm of fullness and emptiness.

Exercising before you eat breakfast also helps sustain a healthy weight. As discussed in the previous chapter, the focus on working your core, glutes and thighs activates acupuncture points that assist in creating calmness, but they are also 'blood building' – they regulate your energy production. If you feel more energized you are less likely to develop cravings for sugary or highly processed foods.

For quicker progress, add nutritional supplements and Chinese herbal formulas to your breakfast. This will boost your energy, prevent cravings and help you maintain a healthy weight. Plant-based Chinese herbal formulas have been used for thousands of years to prevent and treat every symptom imaginable. They flood your body with nutrients, build chi, create chi flow and balance yin and yang so you feel completely and profoundly satisfied.

Gain emotional control

Get your breakfast right and the Peacemaker settles your energy. You'll feel grounded. This keeps aggravation at bay and prevents you from losing the plot during the day, which is bad for your health as well as unpleasant. Instead of being reactive and saying or doing things that you later regret, you'll have the head space to decide how to respond in any situation. You'll spread peace. This is like having a health superpower at your disposal.

What's more, with the Peacemaker working at optimum level, keeping you emotionally balanced, on the ball and less stressed, your immune system will grow stronger and you won't become ill as often. If you do, you'll rebound more quickly. So making time for breakfast will save you having to seek medical treatment further down the line.

Do a clever commute

Add value to this time slot by using your commuting time to your advantage. This is a great opportunity to listen to an informative podcast or audio book, or read something connected to your physical, emotional, spiritual or professional development. This reassures your chi organs that you are moving forward purposefully in this 'drive' time and they will automatically function better.

If you don't have to rush to a job or get kids to school, you can listen to a podcast during your longer walk, or do some inspirational reading (around 30 minutes) at home after breakfast.

UNHEALTHY CHOICES

SKIPPING BREAKFAST

For many people, the morning has become the most chaotic part
of the day: ground zero for the development of symptoms that can
lead to disease. It's a hectic scene of simultaneously checking phones,
drinking coffee, yelling at people to get moving, watching the news,
and munching toast on the run. This combines inflammatory behaviour
with foods that can increase inflammation – the outcome is the rise
of the chronic inflammation conditions that underpin many diseases.

Don't be one of those people that doesn't eat breakfast; if you want
to be healthy this is a non-negotiable meal. If you can't face food in
the morning, it is probably because you have not initiated the detox
phase with morning exercise. If the Cleaner hasn't been able to do
its job, the thought of food can put you off. But skip breakfast and
the resources you need for the day ahead will be drawn from your
own chi reserves. Instead of building chi, you will be consuming chi
and heading into deficit. This leads to sudden energy crashes in
the afternoon, aggravation, listlessness, mood swings, weight gain
and sleep problems. These, in turn, contribute to diseases.

Some people choose to skip breakfast as part of a fasting diet
recommending no food until lunchtime and a large evening meal.
But the Peacemaker doesn't like this: it doesn't build chi, so the
Peacemaker can't spread chi. Then it can't generate energy,
and it can't convert fat into energy. Combine a morning fast with
a large evening meal and you have one of the causes of belly fat.
The chi cycle routine already delivers a natural, organ-friendly
fast of around 12 hours between the evening meal and breakfast.
If you want a longer fast, it is better to skip dinner than breakfast.

Stomach symptoms
Trench warfare

If you are worked up, arguing, stressed-out about work, listening to bad news, following gossip on social media, or answering work emails while eating, your chi can't flow. You're throwing grenades into the middle of the peace negotiations. The Peacemaker can't do its job and rebellion and anarchy are created.

War is declared. Your stomach becomes a battlefield for digestive problems: acid reflux, bloating and distension. Valuable nutrients are not assimilated by your organs – they are either eliminated (straight down the toilet) or stored as belly fat. Your body becomes increasingly desperate for nutrients and you'll start to crave highly processed foods. These create more stagnation in the stomach and the sugars, fats and toxins infiltrate your blood, clog your arteries and create the conditions for atherosclerosis, Type 2 diabetes, high blood pressure and heart disease.

Our lives might seem to be going faster (this is due to a yang imbalance) but critical organ processes such as digestion can't go faster. The Peacemaker follows the clock, not your perceptions of time, and it needs those 20 minutes to do its work. If you interfere with this it creates disruptions that affect all your organs. The symptoms associated with stomach patterns include: bad breath, bleeding or swollen gums, a dry mouth, loss of taste and loss of appetite, constant hunger, loose stools or constipation, nausea, tiredness and muscle weakness. Changing your breakfast behaviour will help to treat these symptoms and prevent more serious ones from developing.

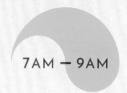
LIFESTYLE TIPS

DOS

Plan your breakfast and prepare it the night before. This takes a potential stressor out of your morning. For example, you could put your porridge mix in the fridge overnight to soak.

Include feel-good grains or carbs in your breakfast, such as oats, barley, buckwheat, rye, brown rice or sweet potatoes.

Add a high-quality protein powder to your breakfast. Protein is essential for healthy skin, muscles, cartilage, bones and blood, and is anti-ageing. It will help stabilize your emotions and keep your energy up until lunchtime, which prevents cravings and snacking.

Change your breakfast menu slowly.

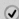

If you are a coffee drinker, enjoy one or two cups after breakfast.

Take high-quality nutritional supplements. These enhance the health of your organs. The basics are antioxidants, minerals, essential fatty acids and a multivitamin.

Sit down while you eat and do your best to create a peaceful atmosphere so that your food can go down. Listening to calming music helps with this.

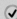

If you only have five or ten minutes for breakfast, still eat calmly with as little distraction as possible. This helps develop life-saving yin skills.

Ban phones from the breakfast table and have all digital devices out of sight. Just seeing these can excite your chi – this feels good, which is why we love devices – but for health your chi needs to sink right now. Excitement comes later.

DON'TS

Eat on the run or skip breakfast.

Drink coffee before eating. Coffee raises your energy and creates a sense of urgency. This interferes with your stomach chi, which wants to ground you. Coffee itself is not a problem, just drink it after breakfast.

Eat cold or raw foods for breakfast. Cold shocks your organs. Your body has to draw on your own chi to warm and 'prepare' the food so that your body can accept it.

Eat highly processed, sugary baked goods or breakfast cereals. These have no nutritional value; the only things they feed are imbalances and pathologies.

Eat while standing up. It will lead to bloating, and energy crashes later on.

Use your phone or reading while you eat. It takes energy away from the digestive process, nutrient absorption is impaired and food can get stored as fat. Yes, you can gain weight just by texting, scrolling and reading while you eat.

Allow jarring radio ads or TV presenters to yell at you. It disturbs the peace.

Scroll mindlessly on your commute. You don't want to be idling or playing games at this time in the morning. It goes against the health rhythm, which needs drive and purpose right now, so it will have a negative effect on your health.

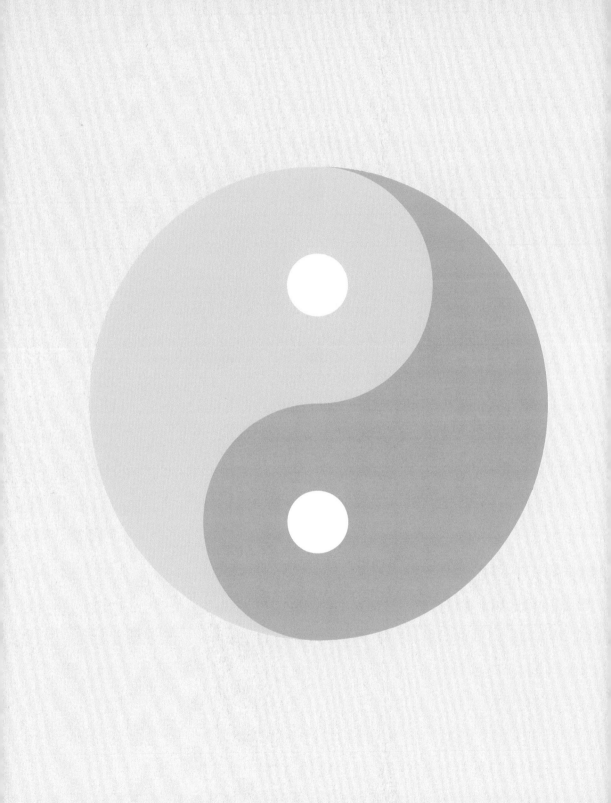

CHAPTER

4

SPLEEN

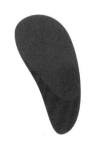

CREATE
YOUR LIFE

From 9am to 11am, your spleen is ready to
build your life. Meet the Builder. This is the
time to work productively.

9AM — 11AM

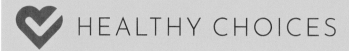

HEALTHY CHOICES

WORK PRODUCTIVELY

The Builder wants to make sure your life has a strong foundation. At 9am it receives a handover from the Peacemaker. The Peacemaker has a grounding energy (yin) and the Builder has a rising energy (yang). So after your calm and collected breakfast, it's time to unleash your mind and work hard. This is the rhythm of health and success.

If you work hard now, the Builder can too. Like hired muscle, it needs to be kept busy carrying materials around, laying foundations and assembling frameworks. The materials it needs are the energy produced from your exercise, the nutrients from your food, and your mental and emotional state while you ate.

A happy builder has just the right amount of work, a clean site, top quality building materials, a clear plan and a great client. To be that great client, go for your goals now, while you are naturally at your most productive (this window extends until 1pm). You'll get more done in less time and have more time for fun later on. This is where work/life balance begins. You are not supposed to be living for work. That would make you unwell.

Lose weight while you work

Working hard at this time of day also contributes to a healthy weight, whereas working hard later in the day or at night can lead to weight gain. If you follow the chi cycle morning routine, your digestive processes will be activated and nutrients are going to be used, not stored. So even if you are sitting at a desk you'll get the weight loss benefits.

The Builder (your spleen) controls muscle, and muscle controls fat. Work hard between 9am and 11am, and the Builder will be busy turning fat into fuel to build your life, instead of into fatty deposits that create symptoms and lead to lifestyle disease.

If you do your part now, the Builder can construct a solid foundation for your life. This helps to keep worry at bay. You'll feel you have a firm grasp on your goals, and the rewarding sensation of moving towards achieving these goals makes you happy. If you are happy, chi flows, and this alone can eliminate symptoms.

YOUR WORK WARM-UP

It is normal to have trouble getting into work mode, but idling and procrastinating at this point in the daily cycle creates symptoms. So, just as you do a physical warm-up at the gym before exercising, do a mental warm-up to mobilize your 'work chi'. Take a minute to acknowledge that you are at work before you begin. It can be as simple as repeating 'I am at work, I am at work' (silently if you are in a busy workplace). Do this even if you work at home, as it issues instructions to your organs. Tap the spleen energy-building acupuncture points below and on the outside of each knee. Tapping these points activates blood and chi flow and stimulates the release of endorphins. It energizes you, enhances your thinking and generates an optimistic outlook. Do two minutes of squats and repeat every hour. Pumping blood into your glutes enhances your focus and clears your head.

Think clearly

In Traditional Chinese Medicine, your spleen influences your capacity for studying, focusing and memorizing. Your organs support brain and body health together, and you need to exercise them both for ultimate health. If you harness your mind to work now it builds a strong foundation for your thoughts as well as your life, and this helps prevent Alzheimer's disease (for the full preventative effects, you need to regularly follow the whole chi cycle sequence).

If you are retired or don't have a paid job it is still important to be working productively at this time of day. Your spleen doesn't care about the pay, it cares about what you do now. You could set up a workspace in your home, write your goals and focus on progressing towards them until lunchtime. Get involved with a cause that is meaningful to you and join a community group, as face-to-face contact is good for your health. If you can't find one, join an online group or forum. All your organs will function better and you will be taking control of your health.

UNHEALTHY CHOICES

Overwork and underwork both harm your spleen. Working hard only benefits you if it is part of a balanced lifestyle that includes rest. If you are 'doing whatever it takes' to succeed, with 12-hour days or 7-day work weeks, you are eroding the foundation of your health, it will collapse and you won't get to enjoy the fruits of your labour. Rest is an essential part of sustainable success.

Underworking

If you underwork and don't challenge yourself, or underperform and clock-watch while you fill in the day at a job you hate, you are making it rain on your building site. Builders hate wet weather and can't work. Because your spleen is affiliated with your muscles, they weaken, are unable to control fat and you will experience puffiness and fluid retention. This is one of the causes of the bulge of flesh around the abdomen and hips in both men and women.

Overworking

If you've fallen into the contemporary lifestyle of being up late at night, waking to social media or working as soon as you wake up, rushing all morning and eating on the run, by the time you get to work you'll be low on energy and more likely to procrastinate, seek distraction, share jokes or gossip, and underwork, just at the time when hard work is necessary for your health. Then you have to catch up by working later in the day or even into the night when your body is supposed to be resting.

You are giving the Builder second-rate building materials and rusty tools. Life becomes unstable. The footings are wobbly, you feel ungrounded and you can't hold your position or establish boundaries. As the tools slip out of the Builder's hands, your goals slip through your fingers. This is what life with an unhealthy spleen feels like.

Your organs support brain and body health together, and you need to exercise them both for ultimate health.

Spleen symptoms
When things fall apart

Underworking at spleen time means you won't have a strong structure for your thoughts and ideas. It leads to short-term memory loss, that unsettling feeling of losing track of what you were saying halfway through a sentence, absent-mindedness, light-headedness and brain fog. These symptoms share many similarities with the clinical manifestations of Alzheimer's disease in Western medicine, and may be its warning signs.

Dementia diagnoses are becoming increasingly common in younger people, and I believe reversing lethargic mornings and overactive nights is the solution. Additionally, poor sleep is a major contributing factor to dementia – people are working late more and more, staying up even later binge-watching entertainment, and then regularly waking to check their phones throughout the night.

The solution is not an occasional 'digital detox', or a rejection of technology, it is to schedule your activities at the times that suit your organs (for social media, this is the afternoon). Bear in mind that everything you do that helps one organ to function well, has an impact on how well the next one can function, and vice versa. Your health will always be moving one way or the other, there is no stasis. By following the healthy choice recommendations in these two hours you are keeping things moving towards wellness, and treating some spleen pattern symptoms like bloating, loose stools, lack of appetite, chest congestion, chills and lethargy.

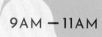
LIFESTYLE TIPS

DOS

If you are a coffee drinker, this is a good time to enjoy one or two.

Make a list of what needs to be done and schedule the hardest tasks of your day now, while you've got full organ backup. Meet the most challenging clients or have the difficult conversations.

If you have a job that requires intense focus, you can support your spleen with Chinese herbal formulas that improve cognitive function and focus.

Exercise your brain.

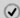

Resist distractions. Switch off notifications on your phone, tablet or computer so you can stay focused. Put your phone away if you don't need it for work.

If you are unemployed, make a list of the things you want to know more about. Divide the list according to professional, self-improvement or pleasure.

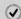

Resolve any relationship issues.

DON'TS

Indulge in social media (do this later).

Gossip. There's never a good time
for gossip – it's bad for your health so,
ideally, eliminate it from your life.

Aimlessly surf TV, video or the internet.
Doing any of these things at this time of
day can lead to immunity disorders and
depression; wait until later in the day.

Retire and just fill in your day with
mindless activities.

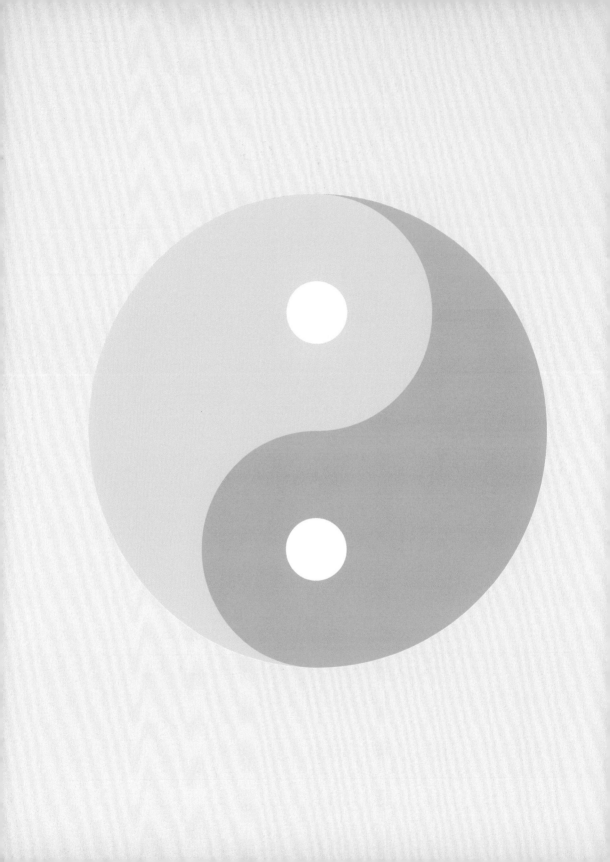

CHAPTER
5
HEART

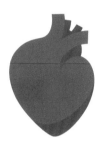

RULE YOUR KINGDOM

Your heart is your most important organ.
It is the seat of your consciousness, the home
of your mind. It is the Emperor. This is the
time to work purposefully.

11AM — 1PM

♥ HEALTHY CHOICES

WORK PURPOSEFULLY

Your heart is a production centre. It needs to be worked. Heart time is the peak of 'drive' time and the health rhythm calls for hard thinking and problem-solving. Your task between 11am and 1pm is both to keep working, and to be purposeful.

You have a mission and your heart, the Emperor, knows what it is. In Traditional Chinese Medicine, knowing and pursuing your purpose is just as important for your health as exercise, diet and sleep. If you feel as if you are on track in life, it enhances your blood flow. This can regulate blood pressure, help prevent the build-up of fatty deposits in the arteries and enhance your immunity.

Your blood carries information, not just about your physical health as it does in a blood test, but also about your emotional, psychological and spiritual health, and your purpose. Work hard now and the Emperor circulates your intention throughout your body so that every time you take a step towards your purpose, it feels 'right'. You become more sure of your purpose daily, and this means you become more healthy and more happy every day.

If you're doing a job that you don't like, still push yourself to work hard, but take a few minutes in this time slot to tune into what you really want to do. You have a heightened awareness at this time. In Traditional Chinese Medicine, life is primarily mystical. There are always unseen forces at work and it is said that the Emperor has access to these and influence in the invisible realms. So visualizing what you want to do can put things into play that will bring you closer to your purpose.

Meaningful connections

The Emperor wants all its subjects to be happy, to feel love, spread harmony and experience deep and meaningful connections with one another. Its job is to support you to be your true self (rather than fitting in with what other people expect you to be). Your organs' task is to support the Emperor in this, and your job is to align with the health rhythm so that they can achieve this.

If you want to talk about any relationship issues, this is a good time to do it, while you have access to reason and your heart's intuition. Relationship issues are often triggered by communication problems, disappointment in someone, concern over their behaviour or irritation with what they say or do. This emotional stress creates organ imbalances and can contribute to high blood pressure, depression, digestive problems and insomnia, so resolution is necessary for your health.

If irritation with your partner is the core issue, you don't even need your partner to solve the problem. When you fall in love, your chi flows freely, which is why everything is blissful. If you later find your partner (or anyone) constantly irritating it is because of chi blockages. The solution is to get it flowing again and a chi practice, such as tai chi, is ideal. This moves chi to all your organs. As each organ presents an aspect of your psychology it is like having a free counselling session. As you practise, it keeps correcting emotional imbalances and, after a while, other people's behaviours won't irritate you. The problem is resolved at the source (you).

This is psychology, chi cycle style. You can also have the 'relationship talk' with yourself; at heart time this can be quite illuminating. And if you do talk things through with your partner, make sure to practise emotional control.

UNHEALTHY CHOICES

If you're slacking off or distracting yourself now, while the Emperor is unrolling the scrolls and revealing grand visions for your future, you are missing an opportunity to improve your health and happiness.

Wasting your potential
You are also wasting the productive potential of the morning and you'll have to pick up the slack in the afternoon and evening. From here on it is easy to lose the rhythm of health and fall into the reverse cycle of working at 11pm and being tired at 11am. But switching 'drive' and 'snooze' has serious repercussions.

 ## Heart symptoms
Trouble at the top

This back-to-front way of living contributes to multiple organ imbalances. These can contribute to heart patterns. Symptoms include: agitation, sadness, confusion, constant worrying, chronic anxiety, impulsiveness, memory loss, postnatal depression, chills, cold hands, tightness in the chest, shortness of breath, palpitations, dizziness, dry mouth, a bitter taste in the mouth, feeling hot and bothered, night sweats, insomnia, lethargy and dark urine.

There are also many psychological patterns in Traditional Chinese Medicine affiliated with the reversed routine. If you're not building chi in the mornings, the Emperor's treasure chests slowly empty and there is no wealth to distribute. Your internal realm is rife with poverty and trouble. You will be susceptible to mental and emotional imbalances and become confused about who you are.

Now it is easy to get caught up in other people's business, particularly family affairs. Your sense of purpose in life slips away, leaving meaninglessness in its wake. You might be lacking inspiration and have no ideas, or you may have too many ideas but can't execute any of them. All these imbalances can contribute to social withdrawal, pessimism and depression.

Meaningful connections to people fade. They become your competitors, enemies – or you just see them as idiots. This leads to dissatisfaction with life, sadness and loneliness. The Emperor wants you to express your true self, but if you can't you'll start subconsciously judging yourself, and in no time become that person who habitually criticizes everything and everyone. People assume that this is your personality, but it's not: it is due to an imbalanced way of living.

This is an impoverished experience of life. And if your life lacks richness, it is natural to seek it outside yourself. It may be through excessive sexual behaviours, comfort foods, cigarettes, drugs or alcohol. These addictive behaviours and substances might temporarily override negative feelings but they 'weaken' your blood, as do all the negative emotions above, and contribute to the development of heart disease.

LIFESTYLE TIPS

DOS

Take a 'chi break' around 11am. If you have a desk job, and have been sitting and concentrating hard for a couple of hours, your blood flow and chi flow have been impeded; you need to get them moving again. Lack of circulation can contribute to high blood pressure, Type 2 diabetes, arthritis and more. The best movement is a few minutes of squats.

If your energy is flagging, have a healthy snack for an energy top-up, such as fruit and nuts, or a nutritious superfood bar.

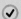

Jot down any ideas you get about projects you'd love to do, or insights into your future direction. If you've been working hard for a few hours you should be in the flow state now, and heart time is when these thoughts start coming through. Keep a notebook or document handy so you can always harvest these thoughts.

If you like journaling, this is the best time for it. As chi flows through your heart in these two hours, you are both intuitive and rational. This is a rare combination.

Talk meaningfully about your dreams and life.

If you can, schedule business planning and presentations in these two hours. This is also a good time to see your bank manager, because you are at your most rational, reasonable and enterprising (and so are they)!

Take nutritional supplements and get energy-boosting Chinese herbal formulas prescribed to increase motivation in the morning and help you to realign with the daily health rhythm.

DON'TS

Gossip. It entangles you in other people's affairs and weakens your emotional control, making you more prone to emotional stress. This creates imbalances in your organs, which cause unpleasant symptoms and can contribute to lifestyle disease.

Drink sugar-loaded energy drinks to perk you up. They don't give you energy, they consume it and you will have an energy crash at 3.30pm. If you are low on energy see a Traditional Chinese Medicine practitioner for Chinese herbal formulas instead, they deliver the real thing.

Slack off. If you're doing a job that you are not passionate about, still push yourself and work hard now instead of distracting yourself with meaningless or entertaining activities. Focusing keeps you aligned with the health rhythm. Your heart houses your mind and you are at the peak time for mental activity. Keep the focus on challenging tasks and your mind won't atrophy.

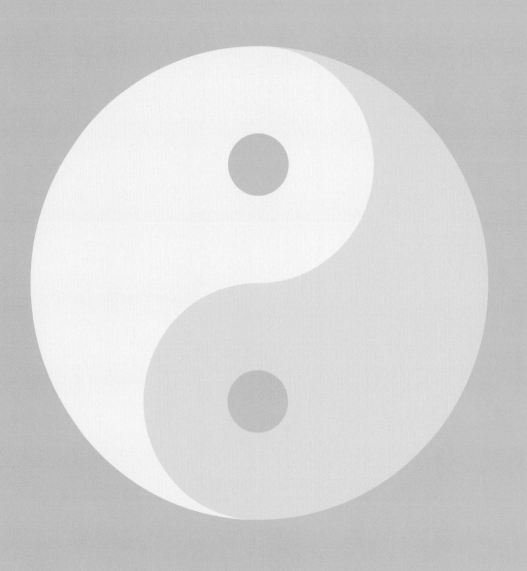

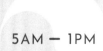 5AM — 1PM

DRIVE SUMMARY

 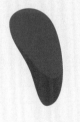 **Get up
and exercise**

 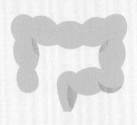 **Eat a nutritious
breakfast**

 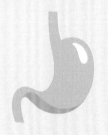 **Work
productively**

 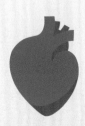 **Work
purposefully**

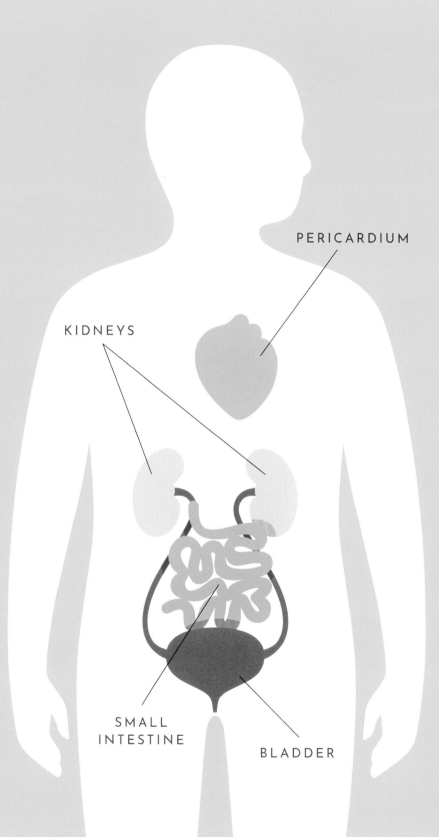

PERICARDIUM

KIDNEYS

SMALL
INTESTINE

BLADDER

2

CRUISE

1PM — 9PM

The yang phase of the day peaks at midday, and now the slow transition to yin begins. Around 1pm it is time to sync with this and start to 'cruise'. If you've followed the 'drive' recommendations over the last eight hours you have been super-productive and have built chi. In the next eight hours of 'cruise' the plan is to reduce the intensity of the way you are working or going about your day. This balances yin and yang and prevents chi stagnation. Don't be misled by the frivolous sound of 'cruise'. Yin and yang imbalances and chi stagnation are the primary causes of lifestyle diseases, including heart disease and dementia. To achieve balance, don't push as hard as you did in the morning. Your organs are ready to take some of the load now. This keeps them in shape and keeps you on the path to health. Now it's time to meet your 'cruise' shift: the Judge (small intestine), Driver (bladder), Puppeteer (kidneys) and Bodyguard (pericardium).

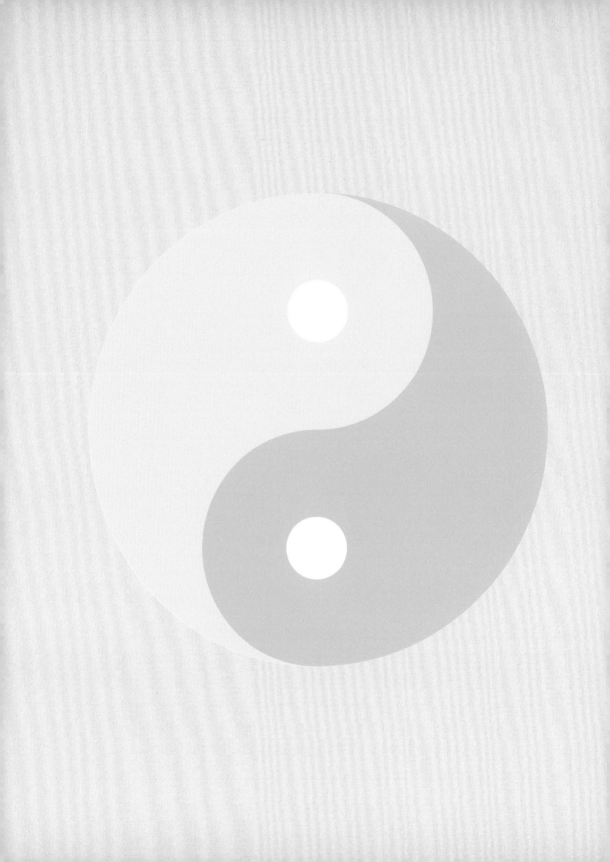

CHAPTER
6
SMALL INTESTINE

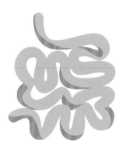

MAKE THE
RIGHT DECISIONS

Your small intestine separates what is 'clean' and useable, and what is 'dirty' or waste. It is the Judge. It is the time to take a lunch break.

1PM — 3PM

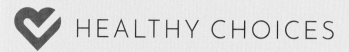

HEALTHY CHOICES

TAKE A LUNCH BREAK

The Judge wants you to make the right choices for health and happiness. Your task is to take a break somewhere around 1pm and have a mindful lunch before getting back into your work.

Mindful eating

Find 30 minutes to slowly eat a nutritious, cooked meal. Acknowledge that you are eating. Look at your lunch. Enjoy it. Savour the tastes. You can even repeat the word 'Yum'. This might sound silly (you don't have to say it aloud), but your organs will get it. Paying attention to your lunch promotes the yin qualities that help you to digest your food, reduce emotional stress and regulate your blood pressure - anything that has this effect is invaluable.

Gain mental clarity and make good decisions

You are before the Judge now. If you do your part by sitting back and having a tasty yin lunch and then return to work while maintaining a calmer state, the Judge can work undisturbed. It will have time to give due consideration to your day's input so far. It can examine your exercise, what you had for breakfast and how much effort you invested in being productive. All your good work (chi, nutrients, positivity) is noted and kept, and anything that might cloud your judgement or have a negative effect on you (toxins, stress, negativity) is sent down towards your large intestine, the Cleaner.

CHI-BUILDING LUNCH IDEAS

An ideal chi-building lunch includes some rice or wholesome grains, vegetables and a protein source. Cold or raw foods, such as sandwiches and salads, are not recommended for lunch. They are what I call 'raw data': although the assembled ingredients might be individually healthy, they have not yet been transformed by cooking into chi. Cold food shocks the body too; it constricts vessels and interrupts digestion. In Traditional Chinese Medicine we use warmth therapeutically to enhance chi flow. Nutrient assimilation is chi (it is described as 'vapour') and eating warm cooked food aids this process, and it means you are working harmoniously with your organs.

Warm meals make it easier to eat mindfully too, because warmth is always nourishing. It gets you out of your head and into your body. If you like cold and raw foods, the evening meal is the best time to have them

If your case is convincing you are awarded mental clarity. This is a fantastic win. With clear judgement, every decision you make is good for you. You'll choose a life partner who is independent and supports your independence, a job that has the perfect mix of challenge and reward, and a lifestyle that prioritizes your health, because you know that without health, nothing else matters.

Help cure insomnia

You might think a lunch break is a waste of time, and that you could be eating while working, but living like this can result in unhealthy symptoms. The upwards energy flow – the yang part of the day – is peaking. The yin stage is about to begin. Working hard all morning and then breaking for a nourishing lunch synchronizes your actions with the health rhythm.

Your lunch break helps establish the yin qualities that will enable you to fall deeply asleep at night and stay asleep right through to 5am. Getting a good night's sleep is how you really gain time. You will wake up refreshed and energized and capable of much more the next day. You'll be super-productive between 9am and 1pm. You won't have to take work home, it will stop dominating your life and take its proper place as one component of a healthy life.

If you don't have a job, are retired or are able to work at home you have a fantastic opportunity to put some extra time and effort into cooking a lunch that nourishes your body, mind and spirit. Nutritious food is the foundation of your health and the Judge will sentence you to a life of health and happiness.

The path to success and happiness is the path of yin *and* yang. Once yang peaks, it needs to shift into yin. Your task now is to facilitate this. Develop the skills of sitting back, slowing down, of spending some minutes after eating doing absolutely nothing. These 'non-actions' will balance yang with yin and you'll feel really good. Case closed!

Put some extra time and effort into cooking a lunch that nourishes your body, mind and spirit.

UNHEALTHY CHOICES

SKIPPING LUNCH

You might think you don't need to eat lunch or you don't want lunch to slow you down. Or, you don't have time to have lunch and would rather be getting on top of your work. But if you do this regularly you will no longer be on top of your health. You'll eventually hand your health over to the medical profession and the pharmaceutical industry. You wouldn't deliberately make yourself powerless in any other part of your life, so don't do that with your health, which is much more important.

If you insist on working through this two-hour time slot, bolting down fast food hunched over your desk or while stressed-out during a meeting, or rushing around multi-tasking with a half-eaten sandwich, energy bar or drink, you are creating chaos in the courtroom and preventing the wheels of justice from turning smoothly.

The Judge is disturbed: it can't apply due deliberation to separate the good from the bad, its cases get mixed up; the good are sent down, and the guilty are free to have a bad influence on you. You will be held in contempt of court for preventing the Judge from doing its work and you won't be awarded clarity. Your decisions become irrational and you'll be much more likely to just fall in with what everyone else does.

Lifestyle diseases are not contagious, but if you are in a workplace where it is the norm to skip lunch, work through lunch or eat while working at your desk, and keep up a relentless pace, and you go along with it, unhealthy symptoms arise. Just because your workmates are heading over that cliff doesn't mean you have to follow them. 'I was just doing what everyone else does', won't hold up as an excuse for organ neglect in the Judge's court. The Judge wants you to make decisions that support your health and happiness. This ultimately serves the greater good.

Poor decision-making and dissatisfaction with life

Disrespect the Judge, and instead of being awarded clarity in deciding what is right or wrong for you, you'll act on impulse. You will make unhealthy lifestyle, business and financial decisions: eat the wrong foods, hire the wrong people, and make poor investment choices. This wastes your time, energy and potential, and it creates unnecessary pain and suffering. It doesn't serve the greater good.

Traditional Chinese Medicine recognizes numerous pathologies associated with impaired judgement, from making hasty decisions you later regret (such as impulse shopping) to an inability to make decisions at all. Either way it leads to feeling dissatisfied with your life and this can trigger compensatory behaviours that undermine your health.

If the Judge can't do its job, chi can't flow freely and by late afternoon you feel stagnant, you've 'had it up to the ears' (your small intestine meridian finishes at your ears). This can trigger aggressive behaviours like road rage, or impulsive post-work bingeing on snack foods or alcohol. Both are driven by an internal need for movement (chi flow) but just worsen the stagnation.

Small intestine symptoms
When your judgment is unsound

If you don't get into the swing of work until lunchtime, which is common, you probably won't want to stop for lunch. Movement is yang, and yang feels good. The problem is that yang creates its own momentum – you feel you have less and less time, and it gets harder and harder to ever stop. The breakfast progression from eating toast at home, to eating it in the car on the way to work (to save time), to swapping the toast for energy drinks is a portrait of unhealthy yang momentum.

If you don't stop and take a lunch break, you are promoting yang dominance and an unsustainable routine. Yang dominance exploits your yin, the quality that is essential for building your blood and for controlling blood pressure, and excess yang contributes to high blood pressure. The quality of your sleep is also directly dependent on yin, so there is a link to sleep disorders and insomnia.

Traditional Chinese Medicine understands death as a complete separation of yin and yang. If your yang keeps rising, your organs perceive a life-threatening imbalance. Your internal alarms go off and your body will be forced into an extreme yin mode, such as depression. You feel unable to move on any level, but Traditional Chinese Medicine sees this as an emergency restorative action to return your body to health. Focus on treating the yang-dominant lifestyle by balancing it with yin.

This will also treat symptoms associated with small intestine patterns such as abdominal pain, bloating, flatulence, stomach rumbling, testicular pain, painful urination, dark urine, hearing loss, throat pain, tongue ulcers, thirst and mental restlessness.

QUICK ENERGY BALANCE

The morning's work takes your energy up into your head.
If you eat lunch in that state it interrupts nutrient assimilation,
creates indigestion and generates unpleasant symptoms.

You can quickly rebalance yourself with a simple chi
practice. Stand with a straight spine as if you are being
suspended from the top of your head. Bend your knees
slightly and hold your arms out in front of you as if you are
hugging a large tree.

Focus on emptying your head and letting that energy move
down into your legs until they feel so heavy they could be stuck
to the floor. Then imagine that you are sending roots down
into the earth. Keep your focus there while you move your
head gently to release tension. You want your head to feel
light while your legs feel heavy but alive. This rebalances
your energy, restores circulation and revitalizes you.

The calming effect of this pose is more powerful than a
tranquilizer. You can use it anywhere and anytime that
you need a quick dose of calm and energy.

LIFESTYLE TIPS

DOS

Plan your lunch and eat at regular times. Lunch and breakfast are the main meals of the day.

For time efficiency, pre-order wholesome lunches for the week ahead, or prepare healthy lunches at home to reheat at work.

Leave your desk or workplace and find somewhere to eat mindfully and in peace. Listening to calming music can help.

Set a healthy lunchtime example for others, especially if you are a manager. This benefits you and your business because it will improve the health, happiness and productivity of your staff. Be a truly visionary leader: make sure your staff take a break and eat a wholesome nutritious meal.

If you catch up with people for lunch, keep it social or celebratory; avoid stress.

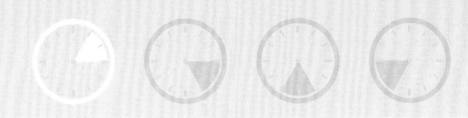

DON'TS

Wait to see what you feel like eating for lunch. Food is way too important for that attitude. It is the fuel for your body, mind and spirit.

Eat cold or raw foods. Your health will suffer.

Use your phone while you eat, even just to text friends or check social media. Just like at breakfast-time, it impairs nutrient absorption, your food is not used and it gets stored instead. This contributes to weight gain, Type 2 diabetes and obesity. If you need to check your phone, text your friends and so on, do it before or after you eat. Switch off all devices while you eat and just concentrate on your food. Try this for a few weeks and you'll notice a significant improvement in your energy and your mood.

Schedule lunchtime meetings or business lunches. If you have meetings over lunchtime that you can't change, still try to leave the office beforehand or afterwards to eat in peace.

Drift along with a toxic workplace culture of eating at your desk. You have free choice. Never eat lunch while working.

Skip lunch or eat on the run.

Drink coffee after 1pm. In Traditional Chinese Medicine, coffee is a herb and its effects last much longer than a temporary caffeine rush. It activates processes that last for hours. The most beneficial time to have coffee is between 9am and 1pm. If you have it later than that, the processes it triggers may create imbalances.

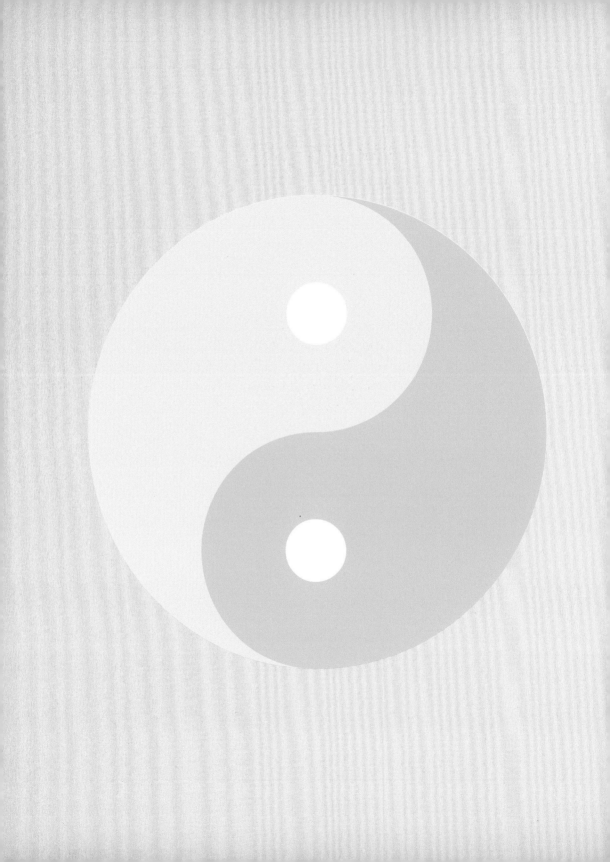

CHAPTER

7

BLADDER

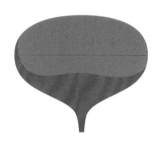

TAKE THE
ROAD TO HEALTH

Your bladder stores the energy you build.
You can catch a ride on that now. Your bladder
is the Driver. This is the time to cruise
through your work.

3PM — 5PM

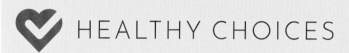

HEALTHY CHOICES

CRUISE THROUGH YOUR WORK

In the afternoon your task is to back off. Keep on working but with a different attitude. Take the pressure off yourself and do the easier tasks of the day. The Driver is ready to take a spell behind the wheel now and if you take the back seat, it can do its job.

Imagine that the Driver is going to be chauffeuring you around in a limo. You've got your laptop, tablet and phone so you can work, but you can also take your eyes off the road, enjoy the scenery and think about where you are heading. The Driver will take you towards your destiny now without you having to push it.

Produce energy while you work

People often tell me that the suggestion to back off at this time of day is unrealistic, but if you follow the chi cycle routine, it is doable. Get the morning 'drive' sequence right, and by now you will have built momentum, made faster decisions, and got more work done in four hours than most people would do in a normal work day.

Behind the scenes this has enabled your organs to do their jobs properly and they've been producing chi all day, even while you were working. The Peacemaker, Builder, Emperor and Judge have converted nutrients from your food, thoughts and actions into chi. The more aligned your routine is, the more chi you build, and your bladder (the Driver) is the main organ involved in chi storage. Now it distributes that chi all along its route, reaching all your organs and delivering blood to your brain so you can work with less effort but more efficiency.

Imagining yourself as a passenger also puts you in a more 'yin' mode. This not only lowers your blood pressure, it helps to conserve your chi. You reap the benefits of vitality, anti-ageing, reduced stress, enhanced immunity, emotional balance and confidence.

Boost confidence and go places
Your bladder meridian runs right down both sides of your spine. It gives you 'backbone'. The bladder is associated with confidence (and its opposite, fear, which is why intense fear triggers urination). If you build and store chi you will confidently take the road to your destiny. Follow the chi cycle and you'll go places!

By the end of the Driver's shift, the satisfaction of a peaceful finish to the day should be coming into view. The Driver drops you off, and the limo door closes behind you with a satisfying click. It feels like closure.

This work-day rhythm applies even if you are retired or not employed. Use the afternoon to learn a craft, a language, a musical instrument or do some other meaningful activity. Your organs are expecting this and the Driver will go the extra mile for you.

The more aligned your routine is, the more chi you build, and your bladder (the Driver) is the main organ involved in chi storage.

✖ UNHEALTHY CHOICES

KEEPING UP A RELENTLESS PACE

If you keep up a relentless pace all afternoon, you are hogging the wheel. The Driver has to sit in the back. You might think you are going places faster or covering more ground, but keeping your foot flat to the floor now uses up more energy than you generate. Plus, you have to focus so hard on the road ahead you'll miss seeing the bigger picture.

The limo stalls and the Driver can't drive you or your purpose. Its chi delivery run is also interrupted, all the organs miss out and a deep-seated emptiness, or the feeling that you are going nowhere in life can overwhelm you. Keep this behaviour up and the afternoon can become the most depressing part of the day.

3.30-itis

From 3.30pm onwards you'll start feeling exhausted or aggravated. A regular energy crash in the afternoon is a low fuel warning. It is so common that it is considered normal, and even treated as a joke in many workplaces. But it is not only not normal, it is serious: it is an indicator that your lifestyle is consuming more chi than it is generating. Your organs can't function without chi, and if you maintain that routine you are accelerating the onset of poor health.

Satisfying 3.30-itis with excessive sugar or caffeine, on top of an overstimulated lifestyle, creates serious yin and yang imbalances that become harder and harder to control. It can lead to high blood pressure, cardiovascular disease and depression. So if you've hit the wall in the afternoon, try wholesome energy-boosting snacks like nuts, instead of chocolate, and green tea instead of coffee.

THE BENEFITS OF GREEN TEA

Green tea refreshes the mind, increases alertness, boosts your concentration and is also an antioxidant powerhouse. It has been used medicinally for thousands of years in China and treats conditions from high cholesterol to atherosclerosis, and it strengthens the immune system. It may also promote weight loss. And there are some delicious blends available.

Bladder symptoms
Asleep at the wheel

Your body contains a high percentage of water, and one of the jobs of your bladder is to store and transform fluids. If yin and yang are not in balance because you are overworking or working too hard at the wrong time, fluids can 'spill over' or become concentrated. This may be experienced as frequent urination, dark urine, a decreased urine output or incontinence.

Other common symptoms indicating that your lifestyle is interfering with the function of your bladder are blood in the urine, a burning sensation when urinating, and thirst. Make the healthy change to more productive mornings and less stressful afternoons and you will treat these symptoms and help to restore healthy bladder function.

LIFESTYLE TIPS

DOS

Schedule less challenging things for the afternoon. This is a good time for routine chores and tasks such as filing, answering emails, stocktaking.

Shift into cruising mode: work with a more relaxed attitude.

If your energy is flagging, take Chinese herbal formulas or nutritious, energy-promoting supplements.

Try green tea instead of coffee in the afternoon. Coffee generates energy, which means it makes your chi flow, but it draws from your own energy stores to do this. Green tea promotes health.

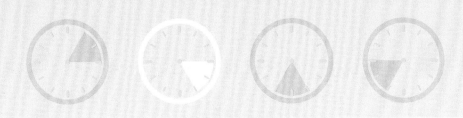

DON'TS

Try to get everything done.
This will never happen.

Schedule important or stressful meetings
for the afternoon.

Give in to caffeine or sugar cravings.
It will interfere with your ability to sleep,
and your 3.30-itis will get worse.

Work hard now. It is against the flow of
the day, and will throw everything out of
sync and create lifestyle disease symptoms.
If you weren't productive in the morning,
do whatever you can to set yourself up for
a more productive morning tomorrow.

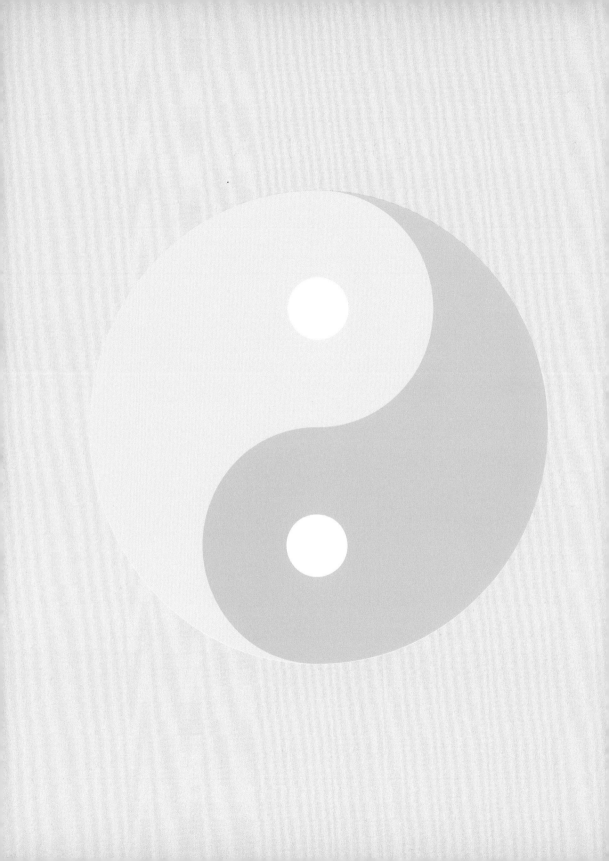

CHAPTER

8

KIDNEYS

PULL YOUR
OWN STRINGS

Your kidneys maintain the perfect balance between
relaxation (yin) and action (yang). They are the
Puppeteer. This is the time to relax actively.

5PM — 7PM

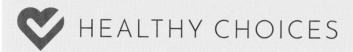

HEALTHY CHOICES

RELAX ACTIVELY

Imagine yourself as a puppet: the 'strings' are your acupuncture meridians, each one affiliated with an organ and an emotion. If the strings become tangled they form knots of anger, frustration, grievances and grudges, and it is hard to feel in flow with life.

People have been jerking your strings all day and throwing you out of balance; this is normal. The Puppeteer keeps your strings moving properly and returns your body to fluid movement. It maintains the balance. If there is too much tension (yang) the puppet becomes rigid and unlifelike, if the strings are too relaxed (yin) it collapses.

Traditional Chinese Medicine sees all disease as the outcome of an imbalance of yin and yang. If this imbalance is not corrected it can progress to a complete separation of yin and yang, which is death. So the Puppeteer's job is critical – it is literally about life and death.

Your kidneys are the foundation of yin and yang for all your organs, so the more you can do to help the Puppeteer do its job, the better. And right now all you have to do is relax for half an hour. No snoozing on the sofa though, relaxation is a technique to consciously transition from being yang to being yin.

Move your chi through your body

Chi practices (yoga or tai chi) are the fastest and most effective means of doing this. Tai chi and yoga teach the art of relaxation, because while doing them you can observe both the process and the outcome of working with the forces of yin and yang. They are self-massage systems too, so you are multi-tasking in a good way.

Every time you do a chi practice, regardless of your level of experience, you are nourishing your organs and mastering the strings. Then, when life gets tangled – as it will – it is less catastrophic because you're in charge of the strings. Loss is less painful, grief and sadness less intense and your life rebounds more quickly to a positive trajectory. Chi practices train you in the skills of the Puppeteer. You will instinctively restore your balance before entanglements can progress into health issues.

A simple mindfulness meditation can also be very effective: the essence is to become cognizant of your feelings and what body part they resonate with. So, take a seat, bring to mind an incident or emotion and observe what part of your body tightens – it could be your stomach, shoulders or neck, for example. Breathe into that muscle until it relaxes. Then breathe confidence and energy into your heart. Let that circulate to every part of your body … you are now disentangling your own strings.

Feel the benefits of exercise

If you usually go to the gym to let off steam or unwind after work, you can use your exercise to disentangle those strings. Bring a feeling such as frustration, fear or anger, associated with something someone said, or did, that triggered you during the day to your mind. Hold it there, merge with it through your exercise, weights or running, and then relax into it. This disentangles the strings.

Access feel-good states on demand

Disentangling enables chi to flow smoothly, which naturally lifts your mood. This helps to reduce the reliance on unsustainable ways to feel good. Sugar or junk food binges, for example, are pleasurable because they initiate a chi flow – but they do so by depleting your chi. The good feelings are short-lived and followed by stagnation. Using these things to change the way you feel can also contribute initially to weight problems.

Other behaviours, such as getting in before the boss, being seen to be busily working through lunch or answering work emails after hours to gain approval (another unsustainable way to feel good) are just as dangerous to your health. There's no point overworking to impress a boss; I'd be more worried about impressing the Puppeteer – it controls the feel-good switch.

You can flip that switch and make yourself feel good at any time with a chi practice, but there is a special quality that comes from doing so between 5pm and 7pm while chi is in your kidneys. You are not in the detox phase, as you are in the morning when exercise requires more effort: this is reward time. Movement feels effortless and the pleasure of chi flow is more intense.

Time for bliss

The Puppeteer is responsible for the interplay between realities. It operates the curtains between the physical world and the spiritual realm. In Traditional Chinese Medicine, both are equally real but for most of us, it is the physical world, where we act out our day-to-day life, that seems most real and feels permanent. This is temporary though, it is what lies beyond the curtain that is eternal. This is the realm of infinite chi.

Practise tai chi or yoga now and the Puppeteer accesses that infinite chi to enhance all organ functions. This is how yoga and tai chi generate therapeutic effects, including reducing blood pressure and alleviating anxiety, depression, asthma, chronic pain, insomnia, and irritable bowel syndrome (as revealed in numerous studies). But chi practices also make you feel really good and this never peaks.

A kidney time chi practice contributes to weight loss too. If your organs are saturated with chi you feel deeply satisfied. All the 'reward-deficiency' triggers are eliminated because your organs have everything they need.

ANTI-AGEING BENEFITS

Your kidneys are also your 'fountain of youth'. If you want longevity and youthfulness, show your kidneys some love. Maintain balance between yin and yang, and keep generating and storing chi. You will look youthful, with optimal skin elasticity, and feel vital regardless of your age. You'll have good bone density so you can remain active and strong; good brain function to keep you learning, growing and engaged; and high immunity for fast recovery from illness. The Puppeteer will keep your movements fluid and supple for life.

No one wants an old age of infirmity or diminished brain function. It doesn't matter how old you are, or how you have been living so far, you can start working on your longevity now. Follow the health rhythm, be conscious of everything you put into your body, and the Puppeteer will keep you running like new. Your kidneys will deliver power, vitality, strong bones, a healthy sex drive and willpower. The chi cycle routine puts you in charge. You'll be pulling the strings for health and happiness.

UNHEALTHY CHOICES

NOT SWITCHING OFF

If you don't switch off, relax or disentangle between 5pm and 7pm, the Puppeteer gets sidelined and the audience, a group of amateurs, are yanking on your strings however they like. The set is collapsing, the script is gone. You are pushed around, your movements are unsupported, life feels threatening, and everyone seems to be against you. Anxiety and fear increase.

If other people pull your strings, your time is not your own and you'll easily become caught up in other people's dramas and their endless demands. You will be more prone to waking up and checking your phone during the night so you don't miss out on anything, and this can quickly become a digital addiction. Your meridians become more tangled, and chi stagnates. You feel increasingly frustrated, cynical and aggravated. You develop self-doubt and feel lost.

You can't see your future and get stuck in the 'good old days' syndrome. You get entangled in the past. Or you become trapped in the idea that you must do whatever it takes to succeed, and work 16-hour days and then get home and collapse on the couch. This isn't relaxation. The couch coma doesn't disentangle. It increases blockages, impairs your chi flow and can contribute to high blood pressure, chronic inflammation conditions or heart disease.

Kidney symptoms
Out of kilter

If you regularly take your work home, or work late into the night, the Puppeteer can't do its job of balancing yin and yang. Maintaining a relentlessly overcommitted lifestyle taxes your kidneys and the foundation for yin and yang for all your organs. Your health will suffer. This is evident in the extended list of symptoms affiliated with kidney patterns. These include: impaired hearing, tinnitus, memory loss, dizziness/vertigo, loss of appetite, loose stools, night sweats, aching bones, sore back, swollen legs, weak legs and knees, lethargy, apathy, dry mouth, thirst and dark urine.

Your kidneys store your sexual power, and a routine that interferes with kidney function also leads to premature ejaculation and impotence in men, and infertility in women. And there's more: healthy kidneys give you your sense of vitality – without it you will look and feel old and tired, with thinning hair, premature greying and poor skin tone.

By now you have probably noticed that many of the kidney pattern symptoms above also appear in the patterns of other organs. Thirst, dry mouth, dark urine, loose stools and lethargy are common. These are early indicators of a separation of yin and yang, and the stagnation and depletion of chi, which are the source of many pathologies and impact on all organs. You can treat your kidneys and target these symptoms every day with a simple chi practice and relaxation technique.

LIFESTYLE TIPS

DOS

Think of relaxation as part of your job.

Finish your work by 6pm, and turn off as many devices as possible that connect you to work. Disconnect properly now and you'll get into work mode faster tomorrow, and be more effective and productive.

Get changed after work. This is as important as getting dressed for work. Whether you change into something smarter or more casual makes no difference. The important thing is to tell your organs that you are no longer in work mode.

Pursue a hobby that takes you away from your daily routine, ideally something creative that you can immerse yourself in. It's a great switch-off strategy.

Do a chi practice to develop your internal feel-good mechanism. This lessens the desire for external feel-good substances that create weight gain or other imbalances. You are never too old to take up a chi practice. You can be in your eighties and it's not too late to start.

Reflect on the day, sit and think or take a walk. Keep in mind that walking is exercise, which is great, but it is not necessarily a therapeutic relaxation activity because you can stay in your head while you do it. If a work or family dialogue keeps running in your head, other people are still pulling your strings.

Take time to enjoy social media, contacting friends, or browsing online.

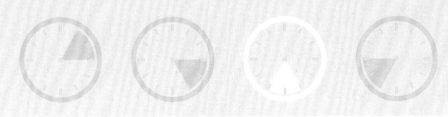

DON'TS

Keep on working past 6pm: this interferes with the quality and length of your sleep, and poor-quality sleep is linked to every lifestyle disease.

Feel guilty about relaxing. Get over this. If you don't develop relaxation skills your health will suffer. If you are a manager without relaxation skills, your business will suffer, as the way you interact with your staff is likely to increase their stress levels.

Drink stimulating drinks such as coffee or tea – even green tea. These will interfere with your ability to relax and sleep.

Go straight from work to a drink to unwind. If you use alcohol to relax you're not pulling your own strings, and that means you're missing an important step in preventing lifestyle disease. Do a relaxation activity first, then enjoy a drink – you'll get the best of both worlds.

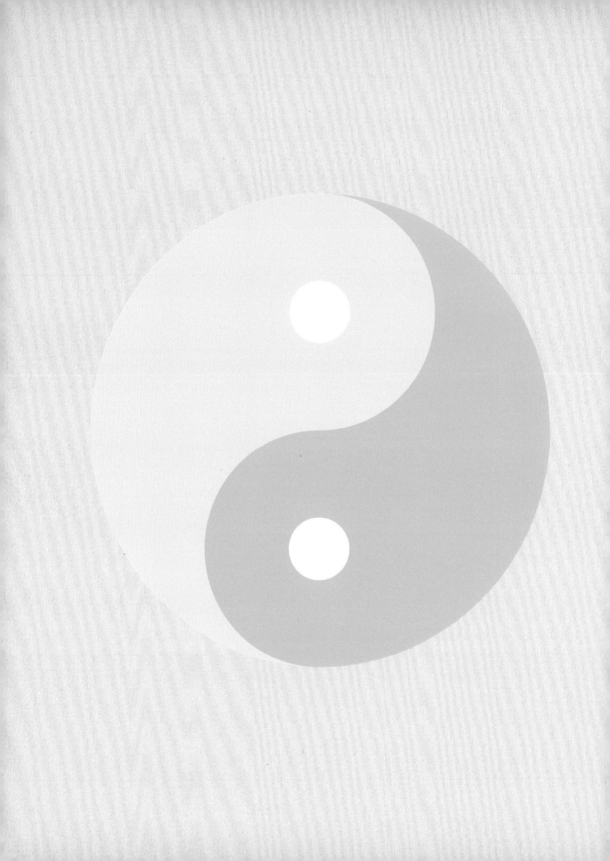

CHAPTER

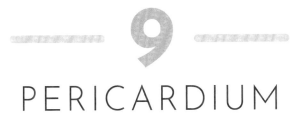

9

PERICARDIUM

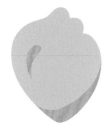

PROTECT
YOUR SOUL

Your pericardium is a membrane that encloses and protects your heart, the Emperor. It is the security detail for your heart and soul. Meet the Bodyguard. This is the time to be joyful.

7PM — 9PM

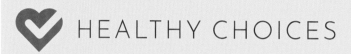

HEALTHY CHOICES

LET YOUR GUARD DOWN

The Bodyguard is also known as the 'envoy of joy' and joy is the expression of your soul. The only business you should concern yourself with from now on is that of your soul.

To be healthy and happy you need to strive to succeed *and* stay spiritually connected. Your normal daily activities – work, business ventures, study, finances and so on are priorities of material success. Your task now is to let that go and give yourself at least 30 minutes to get in touch with your spiritual side. Try to include a bit of joy into your evening.

Joy is spontaneous, but there are also methods you can use to evoke it. Meditation techniques, chanting mantras (otherwise known as the 'yoga of the soul'), ecstatic dance, singing or jamming on an instrument are all mediums of joy. This is not just another daily chore, it is so blissful and soul-satisfying that it becomes the highlight of the day.

Develop healthy relationships

The Bodyguard regulates relationships, because these are matters of concern for your heart. It makes sure you are true to yourself, and it wants you to make heartfelt connections with other people. The Bodyguard plays an important part in feeling joy (falling in love is an example of joy), and protects your heart from the damaging effects of sadness. This is a good time to be with people you love – friends or family who have no opinion on your professional achievements, or lack thereof – and to focus on creating a joyous atmosphere.

Do your part now and you will strengthen the Bodyguard. During the day it will have your back. You will have emotional stability, which protects the health of your heart. With the Bodyguard on side, you'll feel secure in yourself and will be much more likely to have loving and happy relationships.

Many relationship breakdowns are due to neglected and undernourished organs. If you are feeling dissatisfied with your relationship, you might like to think about whether the problem is your partner or your organs (hint: it is usually a combination of their organs and your organs).

Following the chi cycle routine builds physical, emotional and spiritual health simultaneously, so it's an ideal form of non-verbal relationship therapy. If you have issues with your partner, your friends or family, nourish your organs, align with the chi cycle (preferably with your partner). It slowly resolves many of the emotional issues that could otherwise make you stressed and ill, without you even having to talk about them (it's hard to talk rationally if your organs are unhealthy) – instead, each day you both become more emotionally stable, self-assured, independent, purposeful and happy. You'll be on the road to relationship bliss.

Enjoy your life more

Joyful experiences build inner wealth, and the Bodyguard makes sure you don't get robbed of this. As your inner wealth (chi) accumulates, your values shift accordingly. You might put less emphasis on external goals and more on time for yourself and for other people. If you live like this, you reduce your stress levels and improve your health.

You feel mentally and emotionally stable and self-assured and are less dependent on the actions of other people or external circumstances to make you happy. You lose the compulsion to always know what is going on, and to check your phone during the night or to wake up and immediately turn to social media.

You'll be nicer to people, because your soul only knows love. They will then be nicer to those around them creating an epidemic of joy.

The only business you should concern yourself with from now on is that of your soul.

ENJOY SIMPLE FOOD AND SLIM DOWN

Have a light evening meal. This helps you to sleep better and feel better when you wake. Research has shown that a small evening meal is one of the secrets to combating obesity. Your organs prefer a substantial breakfast and lunch, and then a simple evening meal. It is the healthiest way to eat.

A simple meal might sound boring, but as you build your chi, all your senses – including your sense of taste – are heightened. You'll gradually discover richness and depth in simpler foods that you just didn't notice before. At the same time, overly processed, greasy or excessively sweet foods begin to lose their appeal. They become distasteful and finally you instinctively reject them.

This is not something you have to focus on with your mind. Use your mind to follow the chi cycle routine and your organs will handle the rest. Once you are rolling with the health rhythm, communication lines are open and they make the healthy choices for you. You won't find yourself sitting in front of a bowl of kale, looking on enviously as everyone munches pizza! You don't have to battle cravings; you will simply lose interest in the foods that temporarily make you feel good, but then make you feel bad with bloating, indigestion and other symptoms.

The chi cycle routine is the ultimate easy and sustainable weight-loss system, because you build your chi (which makes you feel awesome) and your organs take care of everything else.

UNHEALTHY CHOICES

If you spend these two hours trying to get on top of work (even if you love your job), arguing, being opinionated on social media, looking at images of catastrophic or negative events, watching violent movies with shocking or horrific scenes, or mindlessly channel surfing, you are preventing the Bodyguard from protecting your heart.

If you are out socializing with friends, but focused on your phone or devices, it takes the meaningful, heartfelt element out. If you are torturing yourself with social media images of your exes having fun, or getting envious over happy snaps of friends, or are on social media presenting yourself as happier or more together than you really feel, it's as if you are trying to give the Bodyguard the slip. You're ducking into doorways, changing hats and running down dark alleys. But lose your Bodyguard and you lose yourself.

Unhealthy relationships

You need the Bodyguard on side. It is your closest ally; it provides the backup for healthy relationships with friends and family. If you don't nurture your spiritual side, the Bodyguard can't do its job and you become less secure in yourself. This leads to emotional and mental instabilities and socializing can become stressful. This is how some people can become reliant on alcohol or drugs to feel secure socializing.

Depleted chi and imbalances of yin and yang always go hand in hand with insecurity and can also lead to over-dependence on external security from jobs, relationships or finances. But you can't depend on any of these, true security comes from healthy organs.

If you are missing your daily dose of joy, communications are down, threats are not diverted, security is lax. Blood pressure problems arise and your heart is exposed and vulnerable. Lack of joy becomes a contributing factor to sadness, depression and some illnesses. Without joy fun becomes more important, but it is reliant on external factors beyond your control. If it rains, the waiter is rude or you have a fight with your friends, fun turns into disappointment and frustration.

Pericardium symptoms
Life without joy

Missing out on your daily dose of joy can also set off unhealthy behaviour patterns, such as the urge to compensate with food. If you don't have a chi-building lifestyle you are depleting your chi because there is nothing in between. Life feels unrewarding so all day you look forward to getting home, putting your feet up and having a rewarding evening meal.

Depleted chi leads to a dulling of the senses, including taste, so you keep needing richer or more processed foods to get the rewarding taste sensation and larger servings to make you feel satisfied. This, in turn, can lead to weight gain, obesity and Type 2 diabetes. Overeating is not the cause: this is usually down to an underlying lack of joy and chi deficiency.

The unhealthy lifestyle choices at this time interfere with the function of the pericardium. Its patterns are similar to those of the heart and symptoms include: agitation, anxiety, depression, confusion, irritability, mental restlessness, a feeling of heat in the palms, insomnia and sleep disorders, and relationship problems.

LIFESTYLE TIPS

DOS

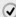

Join a singing group or a dance group.
Do some chanting.

Read your kids a story (children are
great for encouraging people to let their
guard down).

Enjoy some storytelling yourself, as this lets
your guard down. You could watch an hour
of entertainment, or read a book. This is a
necessary intermediary stage between
racing through the day and going to sleep.

Have a romantic dinner with your partner
(this is also the best time for sex).

Turn devices off by 8pm (at the latest)
if you want to sleep.

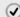

Organize some lunches instead of dinners
for socializing, so you can go to bed earlier
and get more sleep.

See a Traditional Chinese Medicine
practitioner for calming Chinese
herbal formulas.

Practice mindfulness or meditation
to connect to your spiritual side.

Be nice to people. This contributes to your
own emotional stability and happiness.

Immerse yourself in a creative activity
or hobby to leave the day behind.

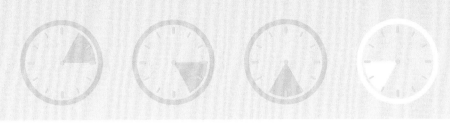

DON'TS

Binge-watch series. After about an hour, this kind of storytelling loses its health benefit and becomes detrimental. Shows are designed with 'cliff-hangers' to keep you hooked, so initially it takes some discipline to watch just one episode. The trick is to get up and move away the minute an episode finishes. It's amazing how quickly that urge to find out what happens next disappears.

Eat greasy, spicy, heavy meals; they will interfere with your organ health and your sleep.

Get back into work after your meal. Avoid even routine paperwork or bookwork – it's still work.

Monitor work emails after hours. You are doing unpaid work and you will pay for it with your most precious asset, your health.

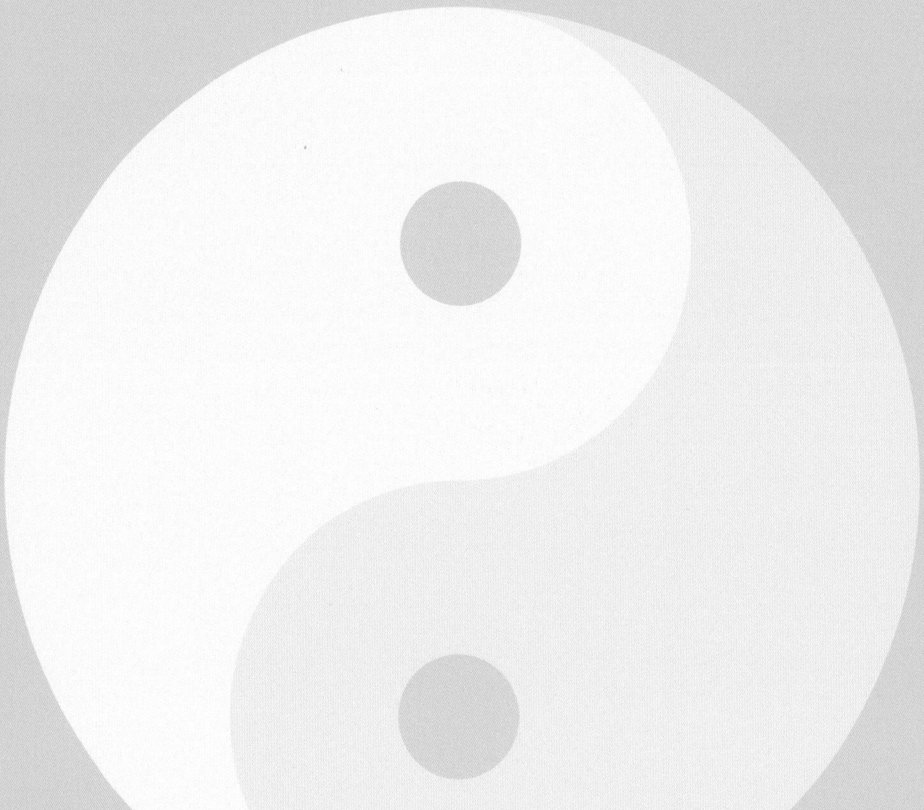

CRUISE SUMMARY

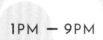

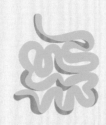

Take a
lunch break

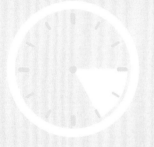

Cruise through
your work

Relax
actively

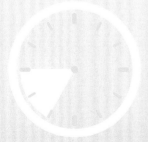

Be joyful

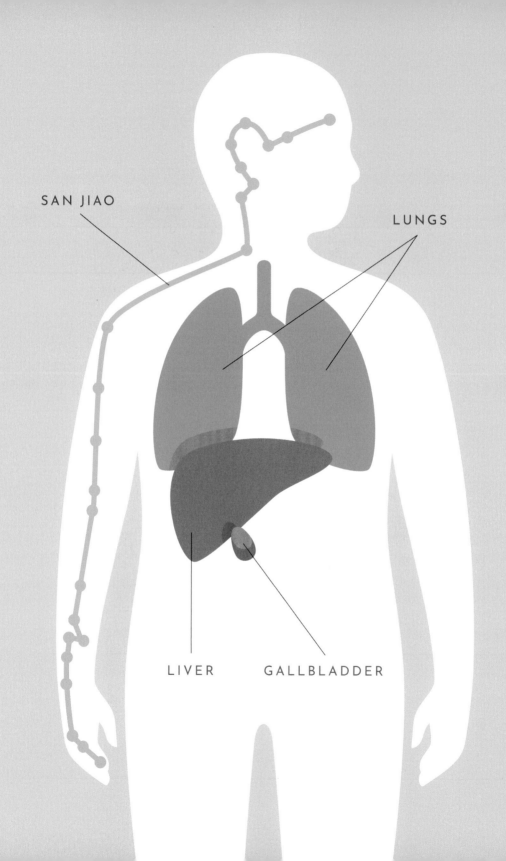

SAN JIAO

LUNGS

LIVER   GALLBLADDER

3

SNOOZE

9PM — 5AM

By 9pm, yin is gaining momentum. If you've followed the health rhythm so far you have done eight hours in 'drive' mode building chi, and eight hours in 'cruise' mode keeping chi flowing smoothly. Now it's time for the 'snooze' phase. This is the most mystical part of the 24-hour cycle. If you sleep, your organs will tap into chi sources beyond the ordinary to heal, rejuvenate and refresh you. 'Drive, cruise and snooze' carry equal weight in creating health and happiness. Sleep is the essential third phase of the health rhythm. It's time to meet your 'snooze' shift: the Ferryman (san jiao), Coach (gallbladder), General (liver) and Knight (lungs).

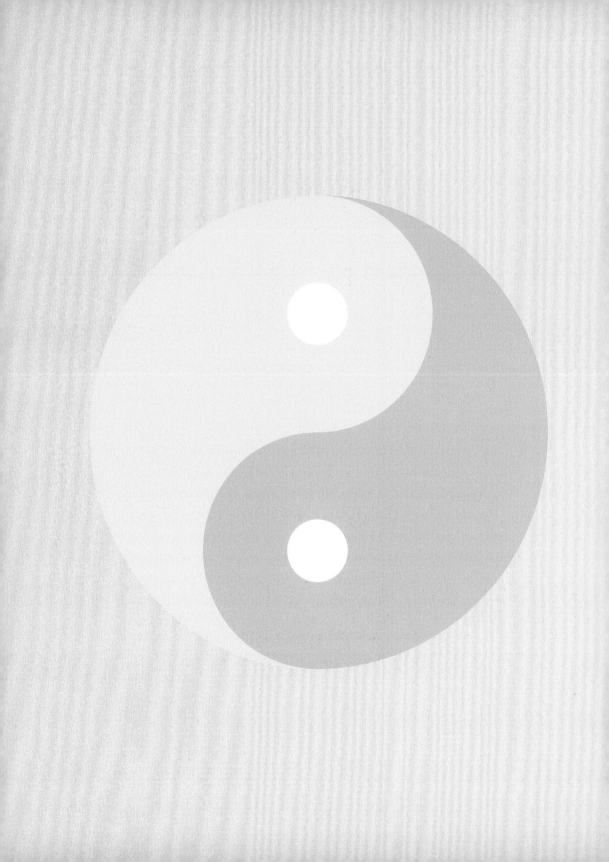

CHAPTER
10
SAN JIAO

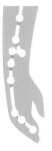

JOURNEY TO
THE MYSTICAL

The san jiao regulates the flow of chi, fluids and
passages between states. It takes you across the
river to the land of sleep. It is the Ferryman.
Now is the time to go to sleep.

9PM — 11PM

HEALTHY CHOICES

GO TO SLEEP

Your task now is to go to bed and hand yourself over to the Ferryman. Sleep is a mystical and complex business – your soul heads back home and your organs get on with maintenance work on your body – and your san jiao is a mystical organ. Sometimes called the triple heater or triple warmer, it is invisible and has no physical counterpart, but its role is essential. It ferries nutrients around and keeps everything flowing so that you get good quality sleep.

There are varying views on how much sleep you need to be healthy, but there is consensus that the quality of your sleep counts for a lot. However, *when* you sleep is also important. Every hour of the day is not the same: they are not interchangeable units, they are each connected to a purpose. The most beneficial hours for sleep are between 9pm and 3am.

I strongly recommend getting to bed at around 9.30pm to catch as much as possible of the most beneficial sleep hours. It takes a while to get into the deeper sleep state, so the earlier to bed the better. It might sound ridiculously early for some people to aim for 9.30pm, but it helps avoid lifestyle disease and capitalizes on the many health benefits of sleep. As with getting up earlier, if you need to make a big shift in your bedtime, make it gradual, say 15 minutes at a time, so your sleep patterns can adjust gently.

Tap into the healing power of sleep

Your san jiao, along with your gallbladder and liver (coming up next), are a specialist health team: they work through the night, every night, to save you from dementia, heart disease, obesity, Type 2 diabetes and more. The deal is that you do your part during the day, and then sleep at night so your organs can work undisturbed.

Sleep is the foundation of health and happiness. Western medicine has found that seven to eight hours sleep a night significantly reduces the risk of both stroke and depression. Traditional Chinese Medicine has found that it increases a sense of purpose and meaning. It is also understood that your organs can perform healing feats beyond normal comprehension. Spontaneous healing and unexpected improvements in conditions that usually progress and worsen can happen while you are asleep.

THE BENEFITS OF SLEEP

Once you are asleep, restoration and recovery processes get underway. Fluids produced by your organs (from your food and drink) are mobilized and distributed by the Ferryman. If you have a healthy diet and take high-quality supplements and Chinese herbal formulas, a nutrient-rich potion plumps up every cell in your body. You wake refreshed and rejuvenated.

Quality sleep, following a day aligned with the chi cycle, creates anti-ageing effects more effective than any product on the market. You don't want to miss this boat!

Catch a ride with the Ferryman each night, get quality sleep, and let the mystical and healing processes of the night hours unfold properly. Your body, mind and soul will thank you.

UNHEALTHY CHOICES

STAYING CONNECTED

The Ferryman keeps things flowing, so at this time your emotions are flowing like water as well. This is why it is common to suddenly feel inspired to talk to your friends, or partner, or get on social media. When I was a drug-and-alcohol counsellor, I often saw young clients who had refused to say a word all day voluntarily start talking about their feelings at this time. Artists, writers, and musicians are often highly attuned to this emotional flow too, which is why they feel they are more creative at night.

This emotional flow is not there to encourage chatting or creative enterprise. If you follow the chi cycle routine and sleep at night, your organs can function properly and you will feel creative and connected during the day. The san jiao emotional flow is part of the mystical chi flow processes that occur while you sleep. Being awake and active now prevents this critical third phase of the chi cycle energy production from happening. You'll be disconnecting yourself from the spiritual mainframe.

Poor quality sleep

Everyone experiences a moment of tiredness around san jiao time – this is the Ferryman talking – but a lot of people push through it to get a 'second wind' and stay up longer. It takes the Ferryman off-course and into dangerous waters; life becomes a struggle to stay afloat, and your boat may even capsize.

You might get by on reduced or poor-quality sleep, for a while, but you won't get the healing benefits of quality sleep. These are only activated if you get to sleep in san jiao time. The thing about insufficient sleep is that you don't see the full effects straight away. The immediate side effects – waking up the next day tired, grumpy or aching – are easy to override with coffee, stimulants or distractions. But the sleep debt accumulates, and when it is called in, the 'interest' makes a loan shark's rates look reasonable.

San jiao symptoms
Missing the boat

The Ferryman stops the health boat running aground by warding off dangers like colds and flu. Go to bed early and you'll nurture and strengthen that defensive function.

The Ferryman can only work with what you give it. Remember that the chi cycle is an integrated system. If you have a healthy diet but don't get quality sleep, you are wasting the potential of the effort you put into your diet. You can drink green smoothies and litres of water all day, but without quality sleep the Ferryman can't do its job properly and the irrigation system malfunctions. The fluid can't enter your cells: instead it is stored around them (fluid retention), manifesting as swollen joints, or a puffy face and neck. Fluid retention is also one of the causes of that bulge around the hips that seems impossible to shake off by dieting.

Other symptoms affiliated with the san jiao include: apathy, body aches, impaired hearing, depression, difficulty urinating, earache, insomnia, loose stools, nausea, loss of appetite, lack of thirst, occipital headache, peripheral oedema, shortness of breath, sore back, sore throat, constant tiredness, weak knees and weak legs.

LIFESTYLE TIPS

DOS

Turn your phone off and go to bed. Leave your phone, tablet, laptop, or smartwatch in another room overnight. Don't look at them or turn them on again until morning, after your exercise. Whatever has happened in the world has already happened, and your health and happiness are more important than any of that.

Chip away at earlier bedtimes: try going to bed even ten minutes earlier at night and getting up ten minutes up earlier in the morning (they are connected).

See a Traditional Chinese Medicine practitioner for Chinese herbal formulas to help you relax and sleep.

Enjoy sex. Another good reason to jump into bed by 9.30pm is that this is one of the best times for sex.

Eliminate light from your bedroom, using blackout curtains.

Keep the TV out of the bedroom.

DON'TS

Keep on working, especially working in bed. This sabotages your sleep – don't ever do it.

Have your phone, laptop, tablet or a TV in your bedroom. Make your bedroom a temple to sleep. because sleep is so important for your health that you should worship it.

Start a relationship discussion late at night (the best time for this talk is between 11am and 1pm).

Fall asleep with the TV on. In Traditional Chinese Medicine sleep is mystical and healing. While you are deeply asleep your soul travels. This contributes to feeling refreshed and rejuvenated when you wake. TVs and electronic devices of any sort interfere with this process.

Take sleep medication. It might knock you out but you won't get quality sleep. Try plant-based Chinese herbal formulas instead.

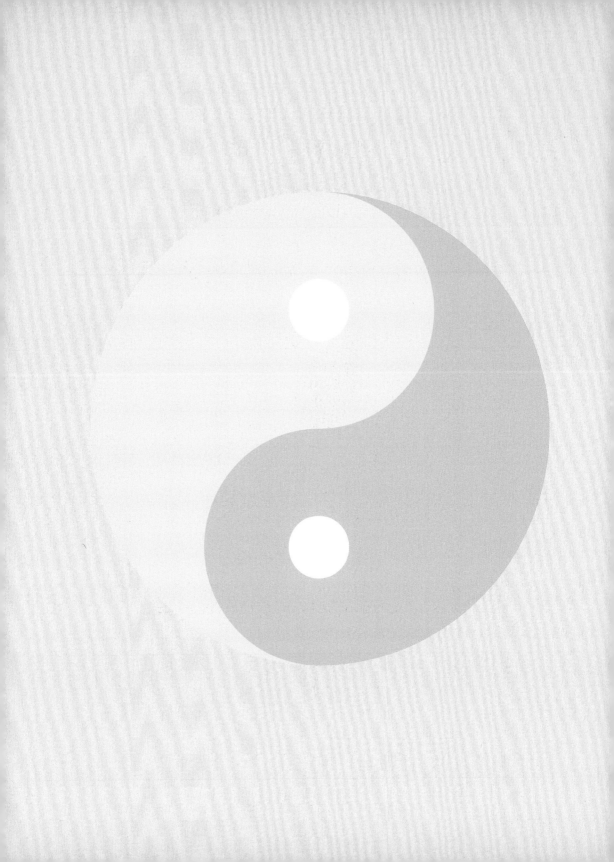

CHAPTER

11

GALLBLADDER

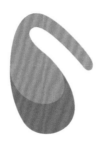

BRING YOUR 'A' GAME

Your gallbladder encourages and motivates the whole organ team to do their very best for you. It is the Coach. Now is the time to sleep.

11PM — 1AM

HEALTHY CHOICES

SLEEP

If you get to sleep by 9.30pm, by 11pm when the Coach clocks on, you should be deep in the land of nod. The Coach can then spend its two hours getting the whole organ team into winning mode. They're all going to be bringing their best game to make sure you can do the same.

Sleeping well

The Coach contributes to the quality and length of your sleep by keeping you nice and relaxed, so you won't toss and turn all night or wake up and interrupt the life-saving work of the night shift. The Coach also supports the smooth movement of your tendons, for supple, flowing movement. Sleep is a great pain management and recovery tool too. This is why most athletes go to bed at 9pm. We might not be athletes, but we can all improve our life performance by going to bed early, like they do.

If you sleep well, in the morning the Cleaner will be extra motivated to do the best job possible, the Builder will be agile and energized, and the rest of the team will be equally inspired to set you on a winning health streak.

Drive positive change and solve problems

Healthy change will also be easier. The Coach carries the spirit of initiative, so instead of just thinking about what you should change in your life – whether that is changing the way you eat breakfast, or changing your job or your friends – you'll be more likely to carry your good intentions through.

You are here to be your best self, and the Coach provides courage for this. It gives you 'the gall' to be an individual. You'll be less likely to develop a lifestyle disease from giving in to social expectations that drain you, or toxic work cultures that contaminate you.

Be asleep at gallbladder time and you'll defy expectations, resist the pull of the mundane and start your own health revolution. Train yourself to get to bed early and to sleep. Coach says, 'You can do it!'

You can give your problems to the Coach too, and it will work with the Judge (small intestine) to solve them while you sleep. This is why the advice to 'sleep on it' works.

Motivation and natural weight loss

The chi cycle is an integrated system in which every action is connected to the next. The focus on glutes and thighs in your morning exercise, for example, activates major gallbladder points. Doing this while the Cleaner is at work (5am to 7am) will speed up your metabolism throughout the day, even while you are at rest. Combine this with sleeping at night, during gallbladder time, and it sets an internal weight control mechanism into motion.

We don't just want the smooth and glowing face of beauty sleep, we want a supple, slim and toned body too, because this means we look good on the inside where it really counts. The Coach is a motivator. It stores and releases bile, which digests fat and converts it into energy while you sleep. So you wake up feeling re-energized and motivated to have a healthy day.

Following the chi cycle routine delivers better weight loss results than dieting and it doesn't trigger emotional imbalances that create the deficiency state and bingeing. The problem with most weight loss diets is that they are based on cold and raw foods (salads and juices), or high fat, meat and no carbs. These eating patterns impair spleen function, which sets off other organ imbalances and chi obstructions that lead to anger, irritability and resentment. The gallbladder function is impaired and fat is not digested, so you diet but end up gaining weight and developing fluid retention (due to spleen). Then fatigue develops, so you do less, burn even fewer calories and put on more weight, leading to even more drastic diets. The yo-yo dieting cycle is now under way.

Dieting is counter-productive. The good news is that you can start a new season of natural weight management wins any time. Get to sleep by 9.30pm as often as possible: you will find it easier to break all the unhealthy habits that lead to weight gain and other symptoms. Your game will improve every day and the odds of a healthy and happy life increase.

You are here to be your best self and the Coach provides courage for this.

UNHEALTHY CHOICES

STAYING AWAKE

Right now, anything except sleep will be bad for your health. But people who have caught their second wind after 9pm often continue to stay awake past 11pm to tune into the Coach's functions, including the spirit of initiative, problem-solving and courage. Some might start writing the report or essay they've been putting off all day, come up with the perfect product, or solve a business or life problem.

The feeling of being empowered to be yourself, another of the Coach's functions, encourages a desire to express your individuality: to dress up and go out. You might have a better body image around 11pm, as your gallbladder regulates your body fat percentage, also encouraging the desire to be out and about. Or you might feel courageous and ready for an adventure. But that feeling of courage can get misinterpreted: it is also common for brawls to start around 11pm.

If you are awake from 11pm to 1am, what you get is basically a 'virtual reality experience'. The Coach is supposed to be building all these assets for you while you sleep, so that during the day you can be yourself, solve your problems, and be motivated to initiate change. By being awake late regularly you are preventing the Coach from doing its job properly, so during the day you will lack courage and initiative and will have difficulty solving problems. Your body image will be worse. Change will seem impossible, and you'll feel you are on your own. It creates resentment.

Of course this doesn't mean never go out after 11pm. Just keep in mind that regularly being awake at that time will have an impact on your health. So, if you find yourself feeling sad, unsure of yourself and generally down during the day, you'll know why. Bring yourself back to balance with Chinese herbal formulas, and by getting as much of your day aligned with the health rhythm as you can.

Impaired decision-making

Many people say they don't have time for seven or eight hours sleep, but sleep is the ultimate time-saver. Not getting enough sleep sidelines the Coach. The team won't be bringing their 'A' game, they will forget the plays, and sooner or later you'll start kicking emotional 'own goals' that sabotage your enjoyment of life.

Your decision-making will be impaired because your internal guidance system is disconnected. You will find yourself doing things that needlessly mess up your personal and professional life, another fast route to resentment. Living like this is the real time-waster.

People also tell me that they are awake at this time because they 'don't need sleep'. This is true for less than one per cent of the population: for everyone else, lack of sleep encourages dementia and lifestyle disease.

Gallbladder symptoms
When you're off your game

The gallbladder can represent a turning point for new beginnings and new stages of life. But this comes down to a team effort between you and your organs. If you're not sleeping at gallbladder time you're not being a good team player. You are throwing off your own game.

You'll be one of those people who are always saying, 'I should change my life, I should get healthy, I should get more exercise', but never get around to doing it. You need to be courageous and make positive changes to be healthy. And for this you need to sleep.

Gallbladder pattern symptoms include: gallstones, blurry vision, dizziness, hypochondriac pain, a bitter taste in the mouth, thirst, nausea, inability to digest fats, dark urine, jaundice, lack of motivation, nervousness, sighing all the time and timidity.

LIFESTYLE TIPS

DOS

Give yourself at least three hours between finishing exercise and sleeping. Vigorous exercise stimulates the yang, which wakes you up and puts you in 'drive' mode. That's exactly what you need in the morning, but to be able to sleep you need to be in 'snooze' mode. If you can't get going in the morning it is because yang is not stimulated, and if you can't sleep at night it is because yin is not nourished.

Give yourself two hours between mental activity and sleeping. Mental activity also stimulates the yang. You can't just turn off the computer or stop work and expect to fall asleep, you need to get your yang down first. In most cases, insomnia is not a medical problem, but a lifestyle problem. You might decide to turn in, but the yang doesn't stop just because you do: it's got its own momentum and it's still rolling. You will need to consciously switch over to yin. Use the kidney chapter strategies, regardless of what time it is.

If you lie down and your mind suddenly starts racing, try a calming sleep tea or Chinese herbal formulas, which can have powerful results.

DON'TS

✖

Watch TV until you fall asleep. Your gallbladder is involved with deep sleep and any screen will interfere with this.

✖

Use your tablet to read in bed – the screen will interfere with your sleep. If you want to read, choose an old-fashioned hardcopy book instead.

✖

Eat spicy and greasy food for dinner – it stimulates yang.

✖

Eat after 9pm.

✖

Add dessert to your evening meal.

✖

Have caffeinated drinks and sweet snacks at night. These stimulate yang and interfere with sleep. If you need a snack, go for a healthy option with no sugar.

✖

Check your phone during the night.

✖

Exercise just before bed.

✖

Work in bed.

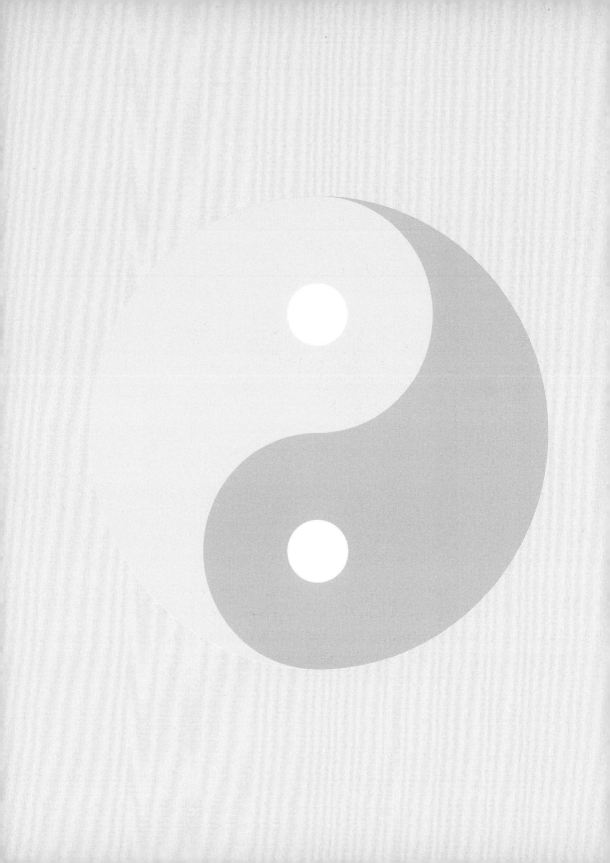

CHAPTER

12

LIVER

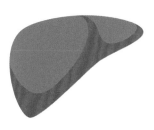

LEAD YOURSELF
TO VICTORY

Your liver is the only organ with its own
authority - its own chi. As it mobilizes and directs
all your organs, and the chi flowing through
them, it is known as the General.

1AM — 3AM

HEALTHY CHOICES

DEEP SLEEP

Moving towards achieving your goals is essential for health and happiness. This is the General's department. The General oversees the execution of your plans. While you sleep, it makes sure you are advancing in the right direction and sends commands down the line to the troops. So when you wake in the morning, your plans are not just conceptual, they have become embodied and more substantial. They feel real.

If you feel resolute you will naturally move towards achieving your goals. Once you make up your mind and act, the General sends in the troops to support you. Your life unfolds according to plan. This makes the General happy and chi flows freely.

Set and achieve your goals

The trick is to keep moving. Your big goal is often so far away it feels out of reach. The chi cycle routine has a nice set of small daily goals ready for you. Think of these as the stepping stones to the big ones.

Achieve these little goals, from getting up a bit earlier to being calm while you eat, and you keep that chi flowing. The General will keep mobilizing and directing the troops and it gets easier and easier for you to plan and then act. Most importantly, get quality sleep every night and you'll keep the General on-side. With an army behind you, nothing can stop you.

Traditional Chinese Medicine is a system of cosmic harmony. Your organs are like small cogs in a much bigger mechanism which connects everything from the micro to the macro.

Your organs don't operate independently: they are under the influence of the General. If you sleep, you support the General to do its job, and it will direct your organs to do their job. You'll be in flow with life itself: healthy, happy and following your destiny.

Take charge of time, reduce stress and be happy

Your perception of time is regulated by your liver, the General. A sleep-deprived, multi-tasking, overcommitted and overworked way of living creates a yang imbalance in your liver. When there is more yang than yin, everything speeds up and time seems to go faster. Life becomes a race against the clock and symptoms arise.

Living in accordance with the chi cycle naturally corrects this imbalance. And, because all your activities are scheduled when they are most effective, you keep gaining time. Getting quality sleep at night rebalances the yin and yang in your liver and time will be on your side.

Following the chi cycle routine won't turn you into a recluse who never leaves home after the sun goes down. Going out is part of life. A fun night out lifts your spirit, and this is good for your health and happiness. The idea is to make your partying occasional, and part of your health strategy. For lots of people, staying up late and going out drinking has become a habit. This has no health benefits.

The General is in charge of happiness. When liver chi flows freely, you feel happy. If you are happy, you are naturally more resistant to illness. Synchronize your life to the 24-hour clock: be up early at the gym, jogging or doing a chi practice. Have a calm and nourishing breakfast. Report for duty and be decisive and efficient at work. Stop at lunchtime, eat mindfully, and switch off from work by 6pm. And be ready to turn in at 9.30pm. Victory will be yours.

UNHEALTHY CHOICES

LOSING DIRECTION

Doing anything except sleeping is not healthy at this time. But it's common for people to be awake now trying to catch up on work, binge-watching shows or socializing and sharing their dreams for their future. The latter feels particularly satisfying because, as the General is involved in planning and direction, the sense that your life is heading somewhere is heightened.

The gallbladder vibe of 11pm to 1am is courageous and expressive, but now – between 1am and 3am – the liver vibe is more personal and intimate. It's that classic scene: late at night around the kitchen table with a bottle of wine and deep and meaningful discussions about life plans. While you talk you feel resolute, you are convinced you are on track in life, and all doubt, fear and confusion is gone.

The next morning though, all sense of direction has vanished along with your resoluteness, and you've either forgotten your plans or feel embarrassed about having shared them. For once, it's not the beer-goggles at work, but an increased awareness of your liver's functions. You have witnessed this function but not activated it. If you sleep instead, the General updates the plans and you activate them by following the chi-cycle 'drive' activities of the next morning.

All talk, no action

We all like to talk about our ideas; it makes us happy because it initiates a temporary chi flow. But if talk (yin) is not followed up with action (yang), it leads to organ imbalances. Habitually staying up late into the night interferes with your ability to act on your ideas, and this leads to unhappiness.

People can get trapped in the talking phase for years and never follow through on any of their ideas. This is a liver imbalance, not a personality type. The best way to correct this, to be able to act on your plans and make your dreams become more real, is to get quality sleep at night and get your 5am to 1pm 'drive' routine in place.

Out of time

Perhaps the most attractive drawcard for staying up past 1am is the feeling of finally having time for yourself. The pressure releases and time stretches out – it is the antidote to the relentless rush of the day. But what you are really experiencing here is the function of your liver to regulate your perception of time.

This is not the healthy way to have time for yourself; you'll have even less time the next day, because you have exacerbated the problem. When you feel you have less time you are under more pressure. You may become short-tempered, and be prone to digestive problems or irritable bowel syndrome (IBS), could feel highly stressed and your blood pressure may rise. You get less sleep to try and get more done which backfires.

An imbalanced lifestyle creates an imbalanced perception of time. If you are always on the go, out of sync with the health rhythm and getting insufficient sleep, it raises the yang in your liver. Then every time you are confronted with something else to do, you'll immediately think, 'I don't have time for that'. It's your liver talking. And what it's trying to say is 'help me'.

Directionless

Clients often tell me that they stay up late because they are 'night-owls'. But Traditional Chinese Medicine doesn't recognize the night-owl type. Unless you've had all your organs and bodily fluids replaced with those of a nocturnal creature, you need to sleep at night. Night-owls usually stay up late as a result of unaligned routines and then it becomes a habit and a preference. Your liver is responsible for direction, so if you don't sleep during this time you can lose your way in life and get side-tracked from your purpose. If you work nights providing essential services to others, it is a very different situation. It is not dictated by personal preference.

THE ANGER CYCLE

If you don't get enough sleep you might feel more short-tempered. This can become a cycle in which the angrier you get, the more difficult it is to sleep. Anger is not good or bad, it is just part of the General's arsenal to use for positive change. Feeling directionless or stuck can create anger. I always ask clients who feel purposeless and angry to describe what triggers them, then ask what they think they could do, say or build better? Even taking small steps towards this will get the troops happily marching along again.

If you don't use anger to implement positive change it forms an unstable munitions dump liable to go off at any time. This might be via impulsive and sudden violent outbursts towards others. The anger is not the issue, your lifestyle is. Don't focus on the anger, you'll just go in circles: follow the chi cycle routine and the General will resolve it for you.

Liver symptoms
In an army gone mad

The General is the only organ that can use its authority for good or bad. You choose which it is by how you live. You can override its instructions by following your own personal lifestyle preferences, but this is the hard road forward. In Traditional Chinese Medicine all your organs are directly under the influence of the General so all disease has a direct connection to your liver. If you have an unbalanced and random routine, you are instructing the General to stage a coup that can topple the Emperor, your heart. If this happens, the troops scatter, surrender, run home or act treasonously. In other words, all your organs malfunction.

Accordingly, the liver pattern symptoms are extensive. They include: abdominal pain, epigastric pain, acid reflux, belching, hiccups, a bitter taste in the mouth, difficulty swallowing, a lump in the throat, dry mouth, dry throat, thirst, loss of appetite, nausea, bloating, stomach rumbling, stomach upsets, constipation/diarrhoea, dark urine, vomiting; swollen testicles in men; amenorrhea, irregular periods, premenstrual tension, period pain, vaginal discharge and/or vaginal itching in women; impaired hearing, tinnitus, blurry vision, eye floaters; anger, depression, fluctuating mental states, irritability, melancholy, moodiness, resentment, unhappiness; insomnia; cramps, muscle spasms, muscle weakness; tightness in the chest; dizziness; nose bleeds; jaundice; brittle nails; sighing; and temporal headaches.

LIFESTYLE TIPS

DOS

Give yourself a two-hour break from your phone, tablet or any form of screen time before sleep. Sleep is a chi activity not a physical activity (which is why you can't force yourself to sleep) and your liver is the main organ involved with sleep. Electronic and digital devices can have an effect on the liver and cause sleep disruption. Symptoms are either difficulty falling asleep, or constantly waking up.

Keep all electronic devices out of the bedroom. Just the sight of them can excite the yang.

If you can't sleep it is due to a stress factor. This is always associated with yang rising and the only way to control this is via your body. Your mind is yang, so if you can't sleep, calmly engage the body. If you lie there feeling frustrated yang rises and it makes everything worse. Get up and slowly walk around putting the focus on your legs. It sounds weird but it activates gallbladder acupuncture points in your glutes that can get your mind back in sync with your body.

DON'TS

Do anything except sleeping.

Eat midnight snacks.

⊗

Check your phone.

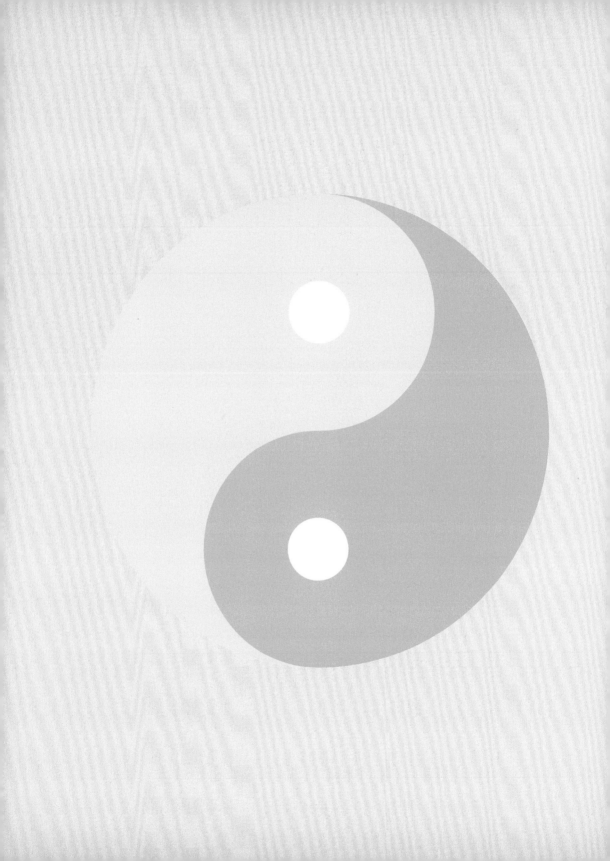

CHAPTER

13

LUNGS

ACT WITH
HONOUR

Your lungs guide you on the quest
for independence and identity.
Your lungs are the Knight.

3AM — 5AM

HEALTHY CHOICES

SLEEP, THEN BEGIN AGAIN

The Knight introduces you to life on earth: with your first breath
you establish independence and make contact with people and
the planet. As chi moves into your lungs at 3am, the Knight starts
a new 24-hour cycle. It is ready to ride as your champion in the day
ahead, supporting your independence and promoting your health
and happiness by ensuring that you act honourably towards
yourself and everyone you meet.

Be true to yourself – and to others

In Traditional Chinese Medicine, the base 'flight or fight' instinct
is controlled by your lungs. As soon as you come into contact with
someone, the Knight fights the urge for the 'base instinct' response
and champions the cause of good by activating your higher instinct
for compassion and love.

The chi cycle routine naturally develops a Knight's code of conduct
that supports this. This keeps the Knight in top shape: fighting fit,
armour polished and sword at the ready. You know who you are,
and you will be protected from any action that might harm yourself,
or others, and lead to ill health. You will be free of the pain of the
past, fully accepting of everyone, and instinctively honourable in
every interaction.

The Knight's job is critical. Contact with people is the major source
of suffering and ill health. If you are suppressed as a child, let down
by your children, abused by a boss or abandoned by a lover or
spouse, it hurts. There are so many ways people can hurt you.
And there are just as many ways that you can hurt others.

When clients talk to me about how they have caused pain in others, the most common things they say are, 'I don't know why I did it', or, 'It's not me'. These statements are correct. It's not you, it is your base instinct. The higher instinct reflects your true self. If you follow the chi cycle, the base instinct won't hijack you and your interactions will naturally be regulated by the higher instinct.

You'll also be able to follow through on any good intentions to change your behaviour. Good intentions on their own are not enough, they need to be embodied – this is the Knight's job. If you live in harmony with the health rhythm, the Knight gets the full backing of the organ team, and will override the urge for revenge or the desire for retribution.

With the Knight keeping the higher instinct as your standard for life, you'll feel good about yourself and will naturally become a 'people person'. You won't blame circumstances, people will rarely disappoint you, you'll lead rather than criticize, and you'll see solutions, not problems.

Embrace change

Your life is a quest for health, happiness and purpose. You want to fulfil your mission. This requires change and mastery of the skill of detaching and reattaching: letting go of the old while embracing the new. Your ability to do this is regulated by your lungs.

As you follow the chi cycle, the Knight's sword is at the ready to cut old ties that no longer serve you. Maybe your friends continue going out every night, and you no longer want to, or your job is eroding your spirit and health, or a relationship has become toxic.

The Knight also supports new connections. The two go hand-in-hand. If one bond breaks, a new bond needs to be formed. If you break up with someone or someone leaves you, the idea is to reconnect with an interest you had previously shelved, or take up something you always wanted to. This keeps chi flowing, which lessens the pain of separation.

Remember to breathe

The Knight works in tandem with the Cleaner (large intestine), so when you wake early and exercise, you are also activating the attributes of the Knight. You can enhance this by paying attention to your breath.

Your breath is the connection between the conscious and the subconscious minds – and breathing techniques are the foundation of chi practices, meditation and all spiritual practices.

Breath can lift you from base instinct to higher instinct. The advice to take a deep breath before you rush into something that you might later regret, works because breath puts you in contact with your higher instinct – your true self. Breathe while you stretch and exercise each morning and you'll remember who you really are.

Your lungs spread chi throughout your body to help all your organs function. The Knight also assists the Emperor in controlling blood circulation. Your soul, which headed off at san jiao time, returns to your body during lung time – bringing with it updated material on your purpose. This is carried in your blood. So exercising early in the morning circulates blood, chi and purpose. Your destiny comes closer with every breath and every beat of your heart.

Save your organs and save the world!

The Knight builds your health momentum. It works with the best of the previous 24 hours to make your higher instinct your default state. This will change the nature of both the contacts you make with other people, and those you make with the world around you.

As the chi cycle reconnects you to the natural rhythm of the universe, you become a better, more considerate and more purpose-driven person. As everyone's purpose contributes to the greater good, this has a flow-on effect, including an increase in the environmental care-factor. Creating a harmonious body leads to a harmonious life, which contributes to a harmonious planet. Everybody wins. This is lifestyle medicine Traditional Chinese Medicine style.

UNHEALTHY CHOICES

HALF-HEARTEDNESS

If you have a random routine, your organ team can't function
properly and the Knight does a half-hearted job. Just as there is
a set of positive attributes that gets developed every two hours
from healthy organs, there is a set of negative ones from unhealthy
organs. The day begins with toxicity, then picks up angst, worry,
meaninglessness, depression, loneliness, fear and grief. Your outlook
changes accordingly. People annoy you and get in your way or
make you sad, angry or jealous. This is the environment for sickness
to develop.

Your lungs are closely associated with your skin: they provide
feelings and sensations. Hence the sayings that people get
'under your skin' or 'give you the shivers'. You get a 'feel' for people
via your lungs. If your organs are healthy, contact with people
generally feels good. If your organs are undernourished, contact
can make you feel exposed and vulnerable. You are not sure
how to communicate, you feel like you don't fit in, you start to
withdraw socially, and then feel lonely and isolated.

Given that the contemporary lifestyle weakens the organs,
loneliness is increasing to 'epidemic' proportions. If the Knight's
sword is blunt, it can't cut off the pain of the past. Maybe your
children leave home or reject you, or your family or partner
stop communicating or move on. You can become stuck in grief,
and isolation or loneliness can follow.

Not letting go

If the Knight can't do its job, you are unable to separate in relationships, have difficulty forming new bonds, or you may turn to a relationship to provide a sense of identity. This is the road to ruin! It may start with the romantic idea that 'He/she brings out the best in me', but when the relationship collapses it turns into, 'Without them I don't know who I am'. This, in turn, impacts negatively on your chi flow and your organ health.

Chi stagnation and deficiencies can cause relationship problems, and imbalanced relationships will erode your health and happiness, often leading to the unhealthy behaviours that generate lifestyle diseases. You might become a people-pleaser and prioritize the demands of your boss, your parents, your partner, your friends, or your children over your own needs. This weakens your chi. Your foundation for feeling good wears away. People-pleasers often crave carbs and sugar: they've been pleasing everyone else all day, so as soon as they get some time for themselves, they reward themselves with a sweet treat, perhaps some chocolate ... or a tub of ice-cream ... Of course this kind of eating can lead to weight gain and many other health problems.

Or you might become a people-hater and start thinking that you are better off by yourself because 'people suck'. I hear this a lot in my work. It is *not* other people that are the issue here, it's your organs. If you constantly talk about not liking people or not wanting to be with people, it is because you are unable to let go of pain or disappointment. Contact with people is essential because it is by interacting with others that you learn who you are. You need contact for your health. If you cut people off, you also cut off the opportunities that could improve your life, as these always come from contact with other people.

WAKING ME UP AT 3AM

A lot of people always wake up at 3am. It is a new chi cycle: chi is entering your lungs, your soul is returning and contact is being made with the physical again. If you are sleeping well, you won't notice this and will naturally wake around 5am. If you have organ deficiencies and yin and yang imbalances, you'll be a 'light sleeper' and the soul's return to the physical can jolt you awake.

The 3am wake-up is the bookend to the 3.30pm energy crash. If you are suddenly wide awake at 3am but haven't had enough sleep by then (at least seven hours a night is the general recommendation), try to remain in bed. Even if you can't get back to sleep, at least your body can get some rest.

If you are still out partying at this time you may be sensitive to the energy shift from 3am. Unlike being awake in the preceding hours, there is no empowerment to tap into between 3am and 5am. Instead the emotions of the lungs can come up and it is common to be consumed by sadness and grief, and just want to cry.

Lung symptoms
When life lets you down

All lung patterns and pathologies revolve around chi deficiency.
The symptoms affiliated with lung patterns include: asthma,
shortness of breath, chest congestion, cough – particularly a
barking cough; constant sweating during the day, low grade
fever in the afternoons, night sweats; dry mouth, dry throat, hoarse
voice, tickly throat, weak voice; insomnia and constant tiredness.

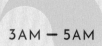

LIFESTYLE TIPS

DOS

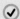

If you are an early riser, follow the 5am to 7am sequence, as your lung and large intestine work together.

If you are up before 5am, you could do more of your chi practice. The more you do of this the better! This is also a great opportunity to add a morning meditation.

Realign with the chi cycle at stomach time, at 7am. Ideally, avoid eating between 5am and 7am as it interferes with the detox phase.

Prevent the 3am sudden wake-up by aligning with the chi cycle.

DON'TS

Wake up at 3am and decide you might as well get up and work because you can't get back to sleep. The only reason you wake up at this time and are unable to go back to sleep, is because yin is not nourished. It is an imbalance of yin and yang. Train yourself to stay in bed until at least 4:30am because your body needs rest to recover.

Think you need less sleep than everyone else because you always wake up so early. It is a symptom of an imbalance, which shows that yang is ruling the yin.

Pull all-nighters for work. This is one of the worst things you can do to your organs. Unless you are a shift-worker or emergency worker, don't do it.

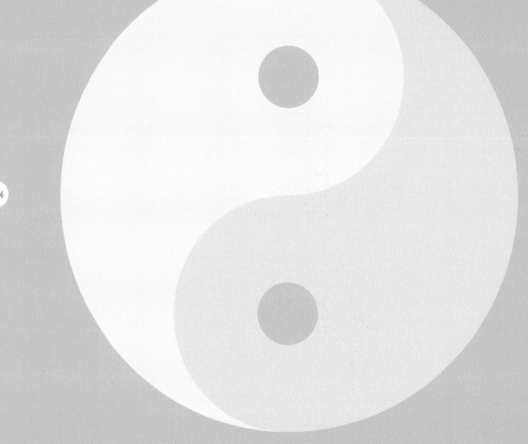

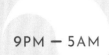

SNOOZE SUMMARY

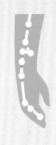

Go to sleep

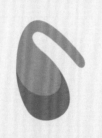

Sleep

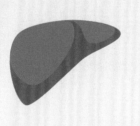

Sleep

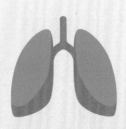

Sleep, then
begin again

CONCLUSION

The chi cycle routine structures your day around a natural rhythm that makes sense for your body and mind. It resets the boundaries between work and personal life, and capitalizes on the potential that every hour holds for self growth, health and happiness.

It introduces a way of living that balances yin and yang, builds chi and enhances chi flow to your organs. This helps to prevent or reverse the imbalances that can lead to hypertension, Type 2 diabetes, heart disease, obesity, insomnia, dementia, anxiety, depression and loneliness.

A chi cycle routine also offers a wealth of emotional benefits. You start eliminating negativity from the moment you wake up. You create inner peace at breakfast, develop strong boundaries and purpose at work, good judgement and confidence in the afternoon, followed by spiritual connection, courage and happiness while you sleep.

With all this under way, your relationships will improve, plus you'll have more energy, slim down, look younger, become purposeful and feel happy. This is a health strategy like no other. It transforms your lifestyle into your best medicine!

INDEX

abdominal problems 34, 45, 78, 139
absentmindedness 55
acid reflux 45, 139
acupuncture points 11, 32, 42, 51, 140
ageing 36, 85, 95, 117
agitation 62, 107
alcohol 63, 77, 99, 106
alertness 87
Alzheimer's disease 6, 52
anger 93, 126, 138, 139
anxiety 6, 7, 31, 33, 62, 94, 96, 107, 156
apathy 97, 119
appetite loss 34, 45, 55, 97, 119, 139
arthritis 64
asthma 94, 151
atherosclerosis 45, 87

bedroom 120
bedtimes 120
belching 139
bile 125
bladder 16, 21, 68, 83-9
bloating 45, 55, 78, 139
blood flow 11, 31, 60, 64
blood pressure 8, 31, 45, 60, 61, 64, 72, 78,
    85, 86, 94, 96, 107, 137, 156
Bodyguard see pericardium
bones 95, 97
bowel movements 30
brain function 55, 95
breakfast 40-1, 44, 46, 47, 67
breath problems 22, 45, 62, 119, 151
breathing 93, 146
Builder see spleen
business management 64, 80, 81, 89, 99

calmness 32, 42, 46
change, embracing 145-6

chest problems 55, 62, 139, 151
chi 10, 84, 94, 107, 151
    flow 7, 10, 16, 73, 93
    stagnation 7, 18, 24, 77, 94, 96, 149
chi practices 11, 36, 92-3, 98, 152;
    see also energy balance pose;
    tai chi and yoga
chills 55, 62
cholesterol 31, 87
Cleaner see large intestine
Coach see gallbladder
coffee 8, 33, 46, 47, 56, 81, 86, 88, 99
colds and flu 119
commuting 43, 47
concentration 87
confidence 32, 33, 85
confusion 62, 107
connectedness 118
constipation 30, 34, 45, 139
coughs 151
courage 125, 129
cramps 139
cravings 45, 46, 89, 149
Cruise phase (1pm-9pm) 18, 19, 69-111
cynicism 96

death 78, 92
decision-making 72, 76, 77, 128
dementia 6, 55, 117, 128, 156
depression 6, 7, 31, 32, 33, 61, 62, 63, 78,
    86, 94, 107, 117, 119, 139, 156
devices, digital and electronic 36, 46, 81,
    84, 98, 106, 108, 121, 140; see also
    phones and TV
diabetes, Type 2 6, 31, 34, 36, 45, 64, 81,
    107, 117, 156
diarrhoea 34, 139
diets, weight control 44, 126

digestion 40, 61, 72
direction, losing 136-8
dissatisfaction with life 63, 77
dizziness 62, 97, 129, 139
drinks see alcohol; coffee; energy drinks;
    green tea; sleep tea and water
Drive phase (5am-1pm) 18, 19, 27-67
Driver see bladder
drug addiction 7, 63, 106

earache 119
emotional balance 43, 85
emotional flow 118
emotional stress 65
Emperor see heart
endorphins 51
energy balance pose 79
energy crash at 3.30pm 44, 86, 89, 150
energy drinks 65
entertainment binge-watching 55, 109
evening meal 44, 105
exercise 7, 8, 30, 31, 36, 37, 42, 67, 93, 98,
    130, 131
exhaustion 86
eye floaters 139

fear 85, 93, 96
Ferryman see san jiao
fever 151
flatulence 78
fluid retention 53, 119
food 7, 22, 86
    cold and raw 22, 73, 81
    desserts 131
    fatty and spicy 22, 109, 131
    see also breakfast; lunch and
    evening meal
frustration 93, 96

gallbladder 16, 21, 112, 123-31
General see liver
getting up 30, 67, 144
gossip 45, 53, 57, 65
green tea 86, 87, 88, 99
grief 148, 150
gums 45

half-heartedness 148-9
hand temperature 62, 107
happiness 6, 7, 8, 14, 15, 16, 18, 25, 74-5,
    95, 108, 117, 120, 135, 145, 156
headaches 119, 139
healing
    and organs 14-17
    and sleep 116-17
healthy choices
    for bladder/3pm-5pm 84-5, 88
    for gallbladder/11pm-1am 124-6,
        130
    for heart/11am-1pm 60-1, 64
    for kidneys/5pm-7pm 92-5, 98
    for large intestine/5am-7am 30-2,
        36
    for liver/1am-3am 134-5, 140
    for lungs/3am-5am 144-7, 152
    for pericardium/7pm-9pm 102-5,
        108
    for san jiao/9pm-11pm 116-17, 120
    for small intestine/1pm-3pm 72-5, 80
    for spleen/9am-11am 50-2, 56
    for stomach/7am-9am 40-3, 46
hearing impairment 78, 97, 119, 139
heart 16, 21, 26, 59-65
heart disease 6, 31, 45, 86, 96, 117, 156
herbal formulas 23, 42-3, 56, 64, 65, 88,
    108, 117, 120, 121, 128, 130
hiccups 139
hobbies 98
home workers 32, 74
hot, feeling 62
hunger 45
hydration 30, 36

immune system 8, 43, 60, 85, 87, 95
impulsiveness 62, 77
inflammation 44, 96
insomnia 61, 62, 74, 78, 94, 107, 119, 130,
    139, 140, 151, 156
instincts, base and higher 144-5, 146
irritability 107, 126, 139
irritable bowel syndrome 95, 137

jaundice 129, 139
journaling 64
joyfulness 102, 104, 108, 111
Judge see small intestine
judgement, unsound 76, 77, 78

kidneys 16, 21, 68, 91-9
knee problems 97, 119
Knight see lungs

large intestine 16, 21, 26, 29-37
leg problems 97, 119
lethargy 55, 62, 97
letting go 145-6, 149
life planning 37, 64, 134
lifestyle advice see healthy choices
    and unhealthy choices
lifestyle medicine 6-9
light-headedness 55
liver 16, 21, 112, 133-41
loneliness 6, 63, 156
loose stools 45, 55, 97, 119
lunch 72-3, 76-7, 80, 81, 108, 111
lungs 16, 21, 112, 143-53

meditation 36, 93, 108, 152
memory loss 55, 62, 97
menstrual problems 139
mental activity before sleep 130
mental clarity 52, 72, 74
mental problems 34, 78, 107, 139
meridians 10, 11, 31, 85, 92
mindfulness 42-3, 72, 80, 93, 108
mindless activities 57

moodiness 139
motivation 36, 125, 129
mouth dryness 33, 34, 45, 62, 97, 139, 151
muscle problems 45, 139
muscles 51

nails, brittle 139
nausea 45, 119, 129, 139
negative emotions 30, 31, 32, 34, 37
nervousness 129
night owls 137-8
night sweats 62, 97, 151
nose bleeds 139
nutritional supplements 7, 42, 46, 64, 117

obesity 6, 31, 81, 105, 107, 117, 156
optimism 51

pain
    chronic 94
    hypochondriac 129
palpitations 62
panic disorders 7
partying 135
past, sticking in the 96
Peacemaker see stomach
pericardium 16, 21, 68, 101-9
pessimism 63
phlegm 22
phones 36, 44, 46, 47, 55, 56, 81, 96, 104,
    106, 120, 121, 131, 140, 141
problem-solving 124-5
Puppeteer see kidneys
purposefulness 7, 60-1, 63, 67, 117

reading 131
relationships 56, 61, 103-4, 106-7, 121, 149
relaxing 92-5, 98, 111
resentment 126, 127, 128, 139
retired people 32, 52, 74, 85
rhythms for health 23; see also time
    phases, 8-hour and time slots, 2-hour
roles of organs 16, 17

sadness 62, 63, 107, 128, 139, 150
san jiao 16, 21, 112, 115–21
second wind 118, 127
self-doubt 96
sex 37, 97, 108, 120
shift-working 23, 138, 153
short temper 137, 138
sighing 129, 139
skin 33, 95, 148
skipping meals 44, 47, 76–7, 81
sleep 116–19, 124, 134, 141, 155
sleep medication 121
sleep tea 130
sleeping in 33, 36, 37
small intestine 16, 21, 68, 71–81
smoking 6, 33, 63
snacking 42, 46, 64, 77, 86, 131, 141
Snooze phase (9pm–5am) 18, 19, 113–55
social media 33, 53, 55, 57, 98, 104, 106
sore back 97, 119
soul 102, 146, 150
spleen 16, 21, 26, 49–57, 126
staying awake 127
stomach 16, 21, 26, 39–47
stomach problems 78, 139
stress 61, 72, 137
stress management 32, 85, 104, 135
stretching 36
stroke 117
surfing, digital 57
swallowing 139
sweating 151
symptoms 8, 9, 22
    for bladder 87
    for gallbladder 129
    for heart 62–3
    for kidneys 97
    for large intestine 34–5
    for liver 139
    for lungs 151
    for pericardium 107
    for san jiao 119
    for small intestine 78

for spleen 22, 55
for stomach 45

tai chi 7, 11, 61, 94
taste 45, 62, 107, 129, 139
testicles 78, 139
thirst 34, 78, 97, 119, 129, 139
throat 78, 119, 139, 151
time perception 135, 137
time phases, 8-hour
    5am–1pm 18, 19, 27–67
    1pm–9pm 18, 19, 69–111
    9pm–5am 18, 19, 113–55
time slots, 2-hour 20–1
    5am–7am 29–37
    7am–9am 39–47
    9am–11am 49–57
    11am–1pm 59–65
    1pm–3pm 71–81
    3pm–5pm 83–9
    5pm–7pm 91–9
    7pm–9pm 101–9
    9pm–11pm 115–21
    11pm–1am 123–31
    1am–3am 133–41
    3am–5am 143–53
timidity 129
tinnitis 97, 139
tiredness 45, 119, 126, 151
tongue 78
Traditional Chinese Medicine 7, 9, 11,
    14–24, 134, 137, 144
TV 47, 57, 120, 121, 131

unemployed people 32, 52, 56, 74, 85
unhealthy choices
    for bladder/3pm–5pm 86, 89
    for gallbladder/11pm–1am 127–8, 131
    for heart/11am–1pm 62, 65
    for kidneys/5pm–7pm 96, 99
    for large intestine/5am–7am 33, 37
    for liver/1am–3am 136–8, 141
    for lungs/3am–5am 148–9, 153

for pericardium/7pm–9pm 106–7, 109
for san jiao/9pm–11pm 118–19, 121
for small intestine/1pm–3pm 76–7, 81
for spleen/9am–11am 53–4, 57
for stomach/7am–9am 44, 47
urination 78, 85, 87, 119
urine, dark 62, 78, 97, 129, 139

vaginal problems 139
vertigo 97
vision, blurry 33, 129, 139
vitality 85, 95, 97
voice 151
vomiting 139

waking up at 3am 150, 152
water 30, 36
weekends 23
weight gain 8, 34, 81, 107, 149;
    see also obesity
weight loss 8, 31, 50–1, 87, 95, 125, 126
weight training 36
working 8, 50–1, 56, 60–1, 67, 74
    breaks during 64, 72, 111
    easing back from 84–5, 88, 96, 98, 111
    and eating 80, 81
    late working 53, 55, 109, 121, 131, 153
    overworking 53, 86, 89, 94, 99
    shiftworking 23, 138, 153
    underworking 53, 55, 65
    warm-up for 51
worry 62

yin and yang 10, 11, 18, 24, 78, 86, 92,
    136, 153
yoga 11, 94

ACKNOWLEDGEMENTS

I'd first like to thank the massage therapist who, after noting discolouration in one of my ankles, suggested I might have Type 2 diabetes. Even though it was due to martial arts training, I immediately searched symptoms online and ended up on multiple fear-mongering sites which, despite my good health, made me feel anxious and confused. As a result, I was inspired to write a book that could empower people to take charge of their health and happiness with simple lifestyle changes.

Thanks to my wife and writing partner, Kirsten, and to my brother-in-law, Leon Fitzpatrick, for his valuable input and illustration of the meridians. Thanks go to my long-term editor, Helena Bond, who provided substantial suggestions for improving the original manuscript. I'm very grateful for the feedback from readers of early drafts including Phillippa Hodgens; Kylie Fitzpatrick for making 'words work harder'; Ngaire Macleod for her encouragement; and Michele Kane for an analytical overview.

My thanks go to the wonderful team at Eddison Books. Commissioning editor, Victoria Marshallsay, was instrumental in transforming the book; Jim Smith worked on the design and Paul Oakley the illustrations. Thanks to Lisa Dyer and OH! for the finishing touches.

Finally my gratitude goes to the great Chinese physicians of old – especially Sun Simiao, the seventh-century alchemist, Daoist and author of early lifestyle medicine publications – who understood that living is an art, that life is mystical and that health and happiness is our destiny.

Commissioning editor: Victoria Marshallsay
Designer: Jim Smith
Illustrators: Leon Fitzpatrick (page 10) and Paul Oakley
Proofreader: Sarah Uttridge
Indexer: Angie Hipkin
Production: Gary Hayes